HEAL
KIDS
HEALTHY
DIET

Sue Kuivanen

Sue@healthykidshealthydiet.com
www.healthykidshealthydiet.com

ISBN 978-0615752020

Disclaimer: The information and ideas in this book are based upon research available at the time of writing, personal experience and opinion. This book is not intended to be a substitute for consulting with an appropriate health care provider. Any changes or additions to your medical care should be discussed with your physician. The author and publisher disclaim any liability arising directly or indirectly from this book.

Special thanks to Michael, Savanah and my editor, J.D. Roa.

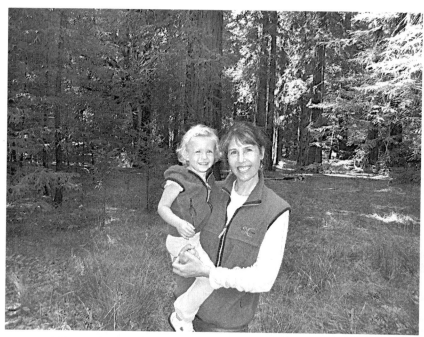

The author, Sue Kuivanen and her daughter, Savanah.

Table of Contents

Introduction

What is more glorious than our children? I love that children are the great motivators in us to achieve, accomplish, and inspire us to be more. We want the best foods and diet for our child's mind, body, and spirit, and we want to provide them with food that's fun and special. We want our children to have a sharp mind and to feel well in their body after eating, rather than moody, hyper, tired, or unable to focus. We want them to be free from sickness and suffering.

Like many parents, I have suffered the pitfalls and anxieties of feeding my child, so it my desire is to address this subject with compassion. Generations upon generations of parents have grappled with how to feed their children, and it has become even more poignant today given the wide variety of food options as well as an increasing amount of food dangers and the terrible health risks associated with our modern diets.

American parents are very much aware of or are even experiencing health crises in their own families such as the rapid rise in obesity, diabetes, tooth decay, autism, and allergies. In just the past thirty years, the rate of obesity has more than doubled for preschoolers and adolescents, and more than tripled for children ages 6 – 11. Currently 17% (or 12.5 million) of children and adolescents aged 2—19 years in the United States are obese.

Alarmingly, obesity is expected to rise to 42% of Americans by 2030, according to the CDC (Centers for Disease Control and Prevention.) The CDC goes on to report that this continued growth in obesity will be very costly to our country; additional spending on healthcare for the obese in the next 18 years is projected to reach $549.5 billion.

As a former English teacher, mother and researcher I have seen the problem of feeding kids well show up in many places – from school lunches, to mixed messages from the media, to the time and money constraints most parents have to deal with on a day to day basis. Add to this the confusing information we get about nutrition and what to feed our kids. There is the low fat diet, the low carb diet, raw food diet, high protein diet, vegetarianism, macrobiotic diet, anti-inflammatory diets, etc. It is enough to make anyone's head spin!

And let us not forget that each child has their own tastes and desires around food. Indeed, it can be challenging to feed kids well and discern "the truth" of what is best for them.

Many of us parents struggle with our own weight and diet, and we don't want our children to grow up spending their lives dieting and battling food-related issues. I once went to an Overeater's Anonymous meeting and heard a woman speak in a raspy voice that she had been battling bulimia for twenty-five years and was fearful for her life. As I listened to her ghastly fate, everything in me cried, "I don't want that for my daughter!"

This is not another cookbook or radical diet program that no human can stick with. Instead, this is a guide for finding balance and moving towards healthier options for our kids, our families, our communities and for our planet.

In this book I provide great ways to get more natural, simple foods into children's diets, tips for shopping, and how to encourage kids to make healthier decisions around food. You'll also find some great kid-friendly healthy snack suggestions as well as encouragement and consolation as feeding your child well sometimes feels like pushing a bolder up a hill. I want you to know that you are not alone in wanting the best for your child and you will find support in these pages.

As you read through this book you'll discover how and why I got involved with school lunch programs and what I uncovered about the "the business of health and food for kids" from school lunches to children's events to shopping for food at farmers markets versus grocery stores. Also provided are the latest research findings about nutrition and vital missing pieces of information about such issues as the relationship between diet and children's teeth, digestive issues and other common health issues.

Just as important, this book is also about opening the dialogue about the relationship between food and health and keeping the conversation going so all of us parents, teachers, caregivers, and food activists can become more informed and help our kids grow up to be happy, healthy, and develop a positive relationship to food. When it comes to nutrition and families, there is no "one size" that fits all, so I have provided you with information, suggestions form experts and various research sources to come to your own conclusion about what's best for your children's health.

I reach out to you with my simple, heart-felt suggestion and share my experience as one mother on a journey with her daughter through a junk food society. I wish on a star that more children can grow in their own gardens and know the deliciousness of fresh fruits and vegetables, feel their bodies grow stronger, and cultivate good nutritional habits that sustain them. I want people everywhere struggling to feed their children, regardless of their various schedules, anxieties, and roadblocks, to say to themselves at the end of the day, with confidence and relief: "I've fed my children well."

Why I wrote this book

There are two important questions this book sets out to resolve: How do I feed my child well and can I and other parents nourish their children well even when we live in a junk food society?

Most of us are aware or are becoming aware of the dramatic rise in severe childhood health issues include obesity, diabetes, tooth decay, autism, and allergies. As early as the 70s, the nutritional advisor to President Nixon warned of an American obesity epidemic. In recent years, the U.S. government recognized a childhood obesity epidemic along with an alarming rise in juvenile diabetes. Less known are the epidemics of childhood tooth decay and adult digestive disorders that start in childhood.

My wish is that this book brings hope, and contributes to new ideas, inspiration, and will advance each caregiver's own understanding for empowering a greater well-being for our children and our communities.

Perhaps the greatest inspiration for writing this book is my daughter, Savanah, who will be six when this book goes to print. I am also a teacher who has taught many ages and subjects in public schools as well as worked with teen mothers, and I have a particular interest and challenge in teaching kids how to express themselves through writing. So I wanted to model that through the writing of this book.

I am happy that my daughter is generally well. I almost didn't have children partly because I was concerned that she or he would suffer with childhood discomforts like I did. Five months before I conceived Savanah, I completed a thirty one day fast. Although pregnancy was not the goal of my fast, I felt my body's house was in better order and I was more confident during my pregnancy about having my own healthy child. I want my daughter to enjoy bountiful health. Being sick is lonely. I don't want children to suffer unnecessarily.

We want the best foods and diet for our child's mind, body, and spirit, and we want to provide them with food that's fun and special. We want them to choose to eat fruits and vegetables. We want our children to have a sharp mind and to feel well in their body after eating, rather than moody, hyper, tired, or unable to focus. We want them to be free from sickness and suffering.

As a child my diet was mainly boxed cereal, maybe oatmeal for breakfast, orange juice from frozen concentrate, 2% milk, cheese, butter, peanut butter and jelly sandwiches, oranges, apples, bananas, meat, potatoes, cooked vegetables, homemade baked cookies and cakes, and store bought ice cream. My family did have a summer vegetable garden. The obvious junk food of candy and soda pop wasn't common in the house. For many of us it feels like a big effort to feed children a different diet than the one we grew up with. It almost feels like changing religions!

The only similarity about my childhood diet and my daughter's is a lot of peanut butter and jelly sandwiches. Except, my daughter's PB&J is organic, no sugar added, and the bread is usually not white. As a kid, my mother served my siblings and I Velveeta because it melted so well for grilled cheese sandwiches. (I'm laughing to myself as I write this.) Velveeta is a highly processed cheese that was heavily marketed on television. I guess some day my daughter will make fun of me for some of the healthy shenanigans I use to feed her. I write about some of these trials and errors in this book: everything from school lunches, sugar, and teeth, to gardening and digestion.

Because so many people are suffering from food addiction and health issues, I am mindful of avoiding using food as a punishment or a reward for my daughter. I also shirk overreacting to certain foods or seeing certain foods as morally bad. For example, meat is not often served at our house but we don't make eating meat evil or wrong. I recall reading somewhere about a doctor running a health sanctuary, and he wrote about how many people show up today with anxiety and fear about eating anything!

Sometimes Savanah gets to the point where she is not interested in any of the food in the house. I sometimes say annoyed: "What do you want to eat?" Her reply is simply: "I'm hungry, now!" I know firsthand that feeding kids well can seem like an unending challenge that continues from one meal to the next.

Some authors point out that feeding children well is still somewhat of a pioneering endeavor; after all, the science of nutrition is relatively new. Or, it may be more accurate that we've totally lost our way. In the Ringing Cedars series of books, Anastasia, the main character points out that there used to not be hospitals, and then very few, and look how many there are today. No one has all the answers. We read books about the nutritional value of certain foods, and the nutrient-depleting nature of other foods. Some books tout the superior value of raw (uncooked) foods, while others tell us that the cooking process contributes to the breakdown of nutrients for better digestion and absorption into the body. It's a challenge for anyone to try to determine "the truth" but especially so for parents.

While this book is primarily about nutrition, it is important to remember that fresh air and exercise are also key ingredients to feeding children well such as the more recent awareness that the majority of the population is deficient in vitamin D. Given the opportunity, it is interesting see how much kids enjoy running and moving their bodies in nature. However, for most parents it is often difficult to get kids into a natural environment every day. The majority of us simply do not live on or near acres of land so arrangements and expenses have to be made in order to get children to parks, farms, and other outdoor adventures. Of course there are those 45-minute karate, gymnastic or dance classes which are great and helpful, but one of the big challenges I see for us as childcare providers is getting daily exercise and fresh air and time in nature.

No matter what our individual dietary differences may be, and parents naturally do have strong feelings about this topic, all of us would choose to provide our children with some fresh whole foods, pure water, exercise, sunshine, and proper rest every day. This is the daily goal. "Some" is the operative word. And in a junk food society, achieving *some* takes effort and strategy!

The challenges as parents in the art of nourishing our children on a daily basis are: one, obtaining and keeping on hand fresh, organic whole foods and clean water; Two, getting our children to eat it; and three, making sure they get time outside and some exercise. These goals may seem obvious and, yet, it has taken much thought and study to come to these conclusions. I have included many practical discussions on how to achieve more of the *some* in children's daily lives.

Because children are growing, their nutritional needs are much greater than the adult. Children's bodies are doing major inside work, like building permanent teeth for a lifetime, so it requires a certain consciousness on our part as parents to keep this in the forefront of our minds. In the midst of driving to and from lessons, homework every night and baseball practice and games every other day we have to make a decision and commitment to ourselves to stay the course with our child's health needs. By focusing on the *some*, children will have important, bottom-line healthy foods, and we can allow ourselves to let go of the rest.

When we step into the remarkable journey of parenthood, a natural motivation occurs within to figure out how we can provide the right foods, environments and opportunities for the needs of our unique family. At this time, we realize how valuable understanding food and nutrition are, but then we may have less time and resources for the pursuit. Along with sharing my passion and study for the art of feeding children well, this book is an account of all the elements that factor into feeding a child within a community and through the school system. Most of all, this book is a fast track for all parents who are too busy to take up the study themselves; a handbook for how to feed your children well.

School Lunch

Background

Two minutes after I finished reading the venerable Jane Goodall's book, *Harvest of Hope*, I got my local school district's nutrition director on the phone. "Do you need some parent support?" I asked. On the other end I heard a woman's enthusiastic and desperate response, "Yes!"

Local Lunches and Parents

Online parent groups can be useful. Because I live in a mountain community that requires parents to drive their kids to just about everywhere, an effective online network helps families to connect with each other locally. I started a discussion about the status of our local school district lunch program online. The fire started by mentioning a concern I've had for a while: "Did you know the school lunch program is serving high fructose corn syrup in the chocolate milk!" Little did I know what I was about to get myself into. I had added, "And just look at the below entrees of one week for the school menu. What are Bosco Sticks?"

Lunch price is: Student $2.75(milk is included) - Milk only price is 50¢

(*) = Alternate Vegetarian

Monday	Tuesday	Wednesday	Thursday	Friday
CHICKEN NUGGETS	CHICKEN TOSTADA	BBQ DIPPERS	ROUND TABLE	CORN DOG
OR	OR	OR	PIZZA OR	OR
(*) "BOSCO" STICKS	(*) "SMUCKER'S UNCRUSTABLE"	(*) BEAN & CHEESE BURRITO	(*) PEPPERONI CHEESE	(*) CHEESE QUESA-DILLA

In response and out of curiosity, one parent looked up what kids eat at elementary schools in Palo Alto, California (a wealthier school district near San Jose, California). She wrote: "Each day they still have hot dogs, chicken nuggets, or pizza –but they also offer a salad w/ wheat roll or similar. Kids pay $3.75 for their lunch. Our kids pay $2.75… Boils down to money, resources, and parents and administration driving change. It's still really shocking for me to see how hampered [we are], and likely a lot of other schools too, by lack of state funding."

Another mom in the group mentioned that she was hesitant to speak up because she worked in a school district. "There are a few things I do know that most people don't," she said. Cafeteria food is a tricky, and even political, business. Most districts have completely different ways of supplying food to students. Her district, for instance, has a contract with an outside vendor. The superintendent made a "money choice," and "though we're fairly well off, the food sucks. It meets the guidelines the state and feds have set up, but I wouldn't eat their food," she admits candidly. Our online community forum is about the only place where she can vent these frustrations to a sympathetic group, parents struggling to raise their children healthy, and still remain anonymous.

There is a father on the group list who fervently follows each post as soon as it appears in the same way emergency road service is often the first to respond. I do appreciate him because he provides a different perspective, often playing devil's advocate. His written response to the school lunch topic was a tongue-in-cheek one: "Another tidbit of reality: I can't speak for everyone out there but I am sure many of us survived school lunches as they were twenty or thirty years ago— most of us turned out just fine."

Parents raised other concerns: their children being picky eaters, the procedures of some classrooms that didn't allow parents to bring their children food, not enough choices. Then there's this whole exploding issue of food allergies and intolerances now that's taking parents by utter surprise and shock who suddenly have to quickly adapt and get educated. One mom's name is Theresa. She had to adapt to special pitfalls concerning her child who is two and a half and suffers multiple severe food allergies, including peanuts (or even someone around him eating peanuts), and is at risk for anaphylaxis (where you literally stop breathing). What upsets Theresa most is that he is allergic mainly to healthy foods because of their protein: peanuts, as mentioned earlier, bananas, peas, soy (which is "in *everything*," she noted), garlic, avocados, sesame seeds, sunflowers, corn, and the list goes on. Consumption of any of these foods listed causes him to vomit, break out in hives, choke, have diarrhea, or stop breathing.

Since many foods are related, it is overwhelming to get him to try a new food to see how he reacts. At one point, he stopped growing and the doctors were looking for other problems like Celiac disease. Theresa considers it a great day when she finds something new for him to eat. After all, "he's a two year old with opinions!" She confesses that it's been a hard adjustment, especially when the family goes out. She was recommended not to eat at restaurants because they have peanuts; cross contamination always puts her child at risk for another allergy attack, possibly one that could prove fatal. Fancy restaurants aren't the only kind of places that put him at danger, but other places, too, that kids can normally enjoy without having to worry about vomiting or breaking out into hives: bakeries, ice cream parlors, various cultural dishes.

"Funny thing is," Theresa noted sardonically in response to a previous post, "he can eat 'crappy' food… Believe it or not, McDonald's is one of the safest places for us to eat when going out in public. Before his allergies, our children had never eaten there. I still cringe, but it's safe. I don't have to sit through a meal wondering if my child may stop breathing. Like [the last mom], I just want to feed my child. It's amazing how much we've had to 'let go' of our healthy desires in order to feed our son. We, his parents, don't have food allergies and he was breast fed for a year, which is supposed to reduce the risk. So when you see others feed their kids 'crap,' there may be other reasons, such as ours. We're keeping our fingers crossed that he will outgrow most [of his allergies] by three. He's already outgrown eggs."

Many parents are disconcerted with the health risks that are involved with sending their kids to school. There are extreme cases, like Theresa's, where the slightest mistake can have long-lasting consequences for her son, and there are other cases, where parents simply want their kids eating healthy foods and not just foods that won't kill them. Deidre, another mom on the board, would later join me in shaping school policies concerning health and school lunches in our area. Inspired by this online forum, she decided it was best for her not to whisk her child away to a school with better test scores and to focus on her local school, "because of the connection with so many wonderful people, including many I have met through this group." Taking her husband's advice, she has stepped up to the plate, vowing "to get involved and try to make things better."

Research and Observation of Local School Districts

I started to research other school districts and reviewed the well-publicized Alice Waters/Berkeley School District accomplishments. I concluded the problem with this model for us is that this project was subsidized by a generous 3.8 million dollar grant from Waters' own foundation. When school officials and others questioned whether her plan was viable in the long run, she responded, "We have to change the paradigm on how we spend money in this country."[1] *What can be done **right now**?* I asked myself. I reviewed Berkeley's published accomplishments.

The Berkeley, California school district accomplishments:

- Salad bars in all of our schools. Organic Salad Bar at the High School
- Removed 95% of processed foods
- Hormone and antibiotic free milk
- Fresh fruit and vegetables served daily
- Almost all food is made from scratch
- All bread and dinner rolls – organic
- All other rolls – whole grain
- 50% of the rice served is brown
- Swipe card systems in almost all of our schools
- 25% of produce is now purchased locally
- All hamburgers and hot dogs– natural and grass fed

---

[1] P.190, School Lunch Politics

First off, kudos to Berkeley that almost all of their food is made from scratch. Not too many school districts can say that today. I wondered why only 25% of their produce was purchased locally since it is Berkeley, California. And if all their hamburgers and hot dogs are natural and grass fed, then I guess they don't use government subsidized meats, and I wondered how they could afford to do that.

I had a teaching position with the Santa Cruz County system many years ago, with a small group of troubled junior high boys. The ferocious appetite and nutritional needs of a boy becoming a man astounds me. I'd watch them wide-eyed at lunch when the food came. The boys grabbed and claimed their food like a pack of wild dogs. In fact, one time I had a fight break out in that classroom, which was our lunch room, and it was over food. One juvenile male took another's lunch and wouldn't give it back. Whenever I could, I'd bring in fresh fruit to help supplement, because the county's school lunch was not enough for their appetite, or the food was too mysterious even for their hunger. I remember the watermelon in particular. They clamored for pieces and displayed the delight one witnesses when a piñata breaks. It was as good as candy to them. One father I know has three teenage boys. He says he feeds his boys with a back hoe.

Once, I subbed at an alternative school where the kids were literally rioting and bouncing in their heavy metal desks. I left promising myself to never go back to that school. A year later it was under new management and I got a position there. One thing that changed was that there was more food available to these junior and high school kids at breaks and lunches. In addition to the lunch program and some school funding, more food was attained by a weekly trip to the local food bank. We didn't have resources to go more often. It was remarkable how the whole school calmed down by the increase in food. I think hypoglycemia plays a major role with this population of kids. They come to school in the morning with their 20 ounce breakfast (an energy drink made of caffeine and sugar) or sometimes a Starbucks caramel and whipped cream coffee. The blood sugar drops an hour or two later, and chaos breaks loose. In Jeraldine Saunders' *Hypoglycemia*, I was struck by one line in particular. The author suggests that low blood sugar may be a major factor in this new generation of school shootings and violence.

There was a kitchen at this same school and funds were allocated for one part time kitchen worker. She prepared and served extra food to supplement the lunch program with what she could get at the food bank every week. When the teenage pregnant moms, and other girls and boys came out for breaks, we had food waiting for them on a couple of carts. It was a school of about a hundred students. Most kids ran to the carts except the oldest who were, in a word, young gangster men. They were too cool for such behavior even though they were hungry, too.

At break, the carts often had some donut holes, scrawny apples, bread and peanut butter from the food bank. Sometimes there would be steamed artichokes. Since we were near artichoke growing country, many students knew how to eat the meat from the skins. At lunch, students would get the district-wide school lunch, a prepackaged and reheated doughy and lifeless pizza slice or hard-to-describe PB&J in an enclosed pocket sandwich. Some of the district lunch foods regularly remained untouched, wasted and after a day or two in the refrigerator, thrown in the garbage. The food from the food bank, on its last days of ripeness and expiration dates, was eaten. Although the teenage diet is well known for the junk, still their young bodies screamed for and appreciated real food.

At this school, I am sure some kids must have brought their lunch and, certainly, kids brought chips and soda, but during the years I was there, I don't recall seeing any students with lunch bags. They depended on that school lunch. After a couple years, new students didn't know, and alumni no longer remembered the asylum days when the school didn't offer food from the food bank. Students started catching some salad dressings with expired labels on them and screamed outrage, "This salad dressing is past expiration! I can't believe we're being served this crap. I'm going to the office to complain!"

Whenever I would survey the kids on what extra programs they would like, the number one thing I heard was cooking classes. We didn't have the staff to offer one. Another real concern with having some of the alternative, gang-related students in the kitchen was access to the knives. Cooking classes (Home Economics) hardly exist in public schools anymore. There are new businesses now for people who can pay and arrange for their children to attend the classes.

Lastly, this alternative school did start a garden and we had a few annual fruit tree planting days. One student wrote, "I didn't want to get my shoes dirty, but after a while I dug in and it was lots of fun." It seems much easier to start farm/garden to school education in smaller schools and bureaucracies.

The creative process unravels the unexpected. I never imagined, nor desired, to find myself in the midst of a local school lunch reform like I am now. Deidre, the mom mentioned earlier who decided to have her child go to the local school and try to make things better, is a nurse and an ergonomist. She accompanied me on a visit to a groovy school on the coast, Pacific School in Davenport, California. We met with the head of their lunch program, Stephanie.

Stephanie started a garden and kitchen program with this elementary school. She prepares lunches from scratch everyday for about eighty students (note: there is a waiting list to get into this school). Stephanie also carries out a program where the elementary students get to come into the kitchen and learn about preparing food, chopping, measuring—something that seems possible only in a small school. While there, I noticed they had a small dining room with blue and white checkered plastic table cloths over the lunch tables and small flower vases on each. It looked inviting and charming.

In Italy, for instance, lunchtime often includes fresh flowers gracing the table. Italy also has a national mandate where all school meals must have organic offerings on the menu, less red meat, seasonal fruit, vegetables, and whole foods.[2] It sounds so civilized and right. And the French children get a whole hour— anything less would be barbaric. I can't imagine that ever flying in the U.S. Our children are generally given about a half hour, which includes standing in line. Below is a glimpse of the Pacific School lunch entrée menu.

---

2 P. 232, Jane Goodall

14

Monday	Tuesday	Wednesday	Thursday	Friday
Clam chowder or Lentil soup	Bean and cheese burritos, rice	Sweet and Sour chicken or tofu with stir fry veggies, Asian noodles	Homemade spinach fettuccini topped with parmesan	Pasta Primavera chicken tenders or veggie tenders

Parents sometimes offer support to teachers but how often do we ask if we can help the school's dining services?

Although numerous health books bring up the importance of good digestion, Russell Mariani in his book, *Healing Digestive Illnesses* (a big problem for many of us), masterfully addresses the need and art of proper digestion. I love this one particular story he tells. His client eats healthy foods, exercises and does all the right things, but she's still having digestive troubles. Mariani spots her one day, driving in the car eating one of her sprout filled, healthy sandwiches and it occurs to him— *how* we eat is just as important as *what* we eat. Since reading that story, I am aware of how I eat at home and while I drive, and it's not pretty. Like a lot of parents, sometimes I eat in the car, at the computer, and while serving food to my child. I want to set a better example. It's another bad habit to break.

Next on our journey, my cohort Deidre and I attended a GO FOR HEALTH meeting that was held at the United Way in our area. It's a meeting that supposedly represents around one hundred and fifty other health related organizations in the area focused on ways to address obesity, but there were only four other people there.

One young woman who seemed like she was in her first professional job after college, worked for the Santa Cruz health department. Her job involved giving a twenty minute presentation on nutrition in underfunded schools, mainly Watsonville, CA, which has large populations of children of immigrant and migrant farm workers from Mexico. She had nothing to report except that she couldn't get into a single classroom because they were too busy having to teach to state tests. These so-called "bad" schools come under tremendous pressure because of their low test scores. Never mind that most of the students speak Spanish at home and in the community at large and hardly hear or speak English until they get to school!

Another woman was an expert in the field of education and nutrition. From her we learned that there's a new federal law that affects school lunches and responds to the rapid rise in juvenile diabetes and obesity. I went home and looked it up.

Section 204 of Public Law 108-265—June 30, 2004

Child Nutrition and WIC Reauthorization Act of 2004

SEC. 204 LOCAL WELLNESS POLICY

IN GENERAL - Not later than the first day of the school year beginning after June 30, 2006, each local education agency participating in a program authorized by the National School Lunch Act shall establish a local school wellness policy.

At this meeting, we received direction for what our next steps should be. They told us to "go back to the school district and ask to see their wellness policy. They probably don't have one."

San Lorenzo Valley School District, Central California

They were wrong about our district not having a wellness policy. If anything, our school district seems weighed down by following all the rules and regulations to the tee. I reviewed the policy that a committee of faculty, parents, and students wrote up in 2006. It was an example of how perhaps a well meaning, sweeping federal law fails at the local level. Here's a glimpse of a policy that doesn't help the lunch program but it meets the federal requirements.

A child nutrition program that employs qualified staff who efficiently serve appealing choices for nutritional foods; that offers a sequential program of nutrition instruction integrated within the comprehensive school health education curriculum and coordinated with the child nutrition program; a school environment that encourages students to make healthy food choices;

People's ideas around health and nutrition vary widely, making these terms almost meaningless. There is nothing in the document about key ideas such as sustainable (i.e.: local, organic, farm-to-school), culture and digestion, gardens, planting trees, or green businesses for students.

The nutritional director, Kimberly, turns out to live less than one block away from me and passes my house every day she leaves hers, while I rarely pass hers, but this coincidence has connected us in a strange way. I should also say that I am so glad Deidre has stepped up to support this effort with me. For one, it's a lot more fun with another person, and two, it's too much of an endeavor to go alone. I organized questions for our meeting.

1. First, explain to us what you mean by your numbers. What percentages of families use the lunch program? How many are on free or reduced lunches?
2. Who makes the food? Where does it come from?
3. What are your top priorities, goals for improving health and nutrition at the school?
4. What might we be gathering and going in front of the board of trustees for?
5. Kitchen staff? Work done for work study by high school kids?
6. Amount of time kids have to eat lunch?
7. Chances of getting recess before lunch for elementary kids?
8. Could we get rid of the HFCS chocolate milk? Would it save us some money?

First Meeting

For a change, my first meeting with our school district's nutrition director, Kimberly, was a meeting I looked forward to and one that surprised me. To make getting together as easy as possible, we met at my house. Kimberly turned out be a quick talker, a smiling blonde with a Virginian accent. First off, Deidre and I learned that the lunch program is losing money, operating at a significant deficit ($100,000 in the red). Kimberly talked at rapid speed: "The first thing we need is to change the lunch fee from 2.75 to 3.00 to not only help with the cost of serving lunches, but to save wait time in the lunch line for making change for kids who come with cash." We talked with Kimberly about how the kids are rushed to eat. She responded, "There's an intense government mandated time constraint to serve lunch within a very short time, and the entire school district must be served within that limited time frame." By the end of our meeting, Deidre and I agreed to first help her with the lunch fee.

After we departed, I noticed how hard it was to communicate with the nutritional director. Kimberly said, she wants and needs to work with us. Yet, because of the hot political bed schools are, she seems careful not to be recorded or to ever respond to us via email. Superintendents and administrations try to please their customers (parents and students) and many times it is over the needs of the teachers. Schools are all vying for students and anxious about keeping their numbers up and their parents happy. Deidre and I are going forth making requests, not demands.

I read a hot off the press book called *School Lunch Politics: The Surprising History of America's Favorite Welfare Program* by Susan Levine. This book shows how lunch programs have been financially struggling all along. Public schools have continuously been yanked by the chain with every passing politician. Schools get bullied at both the federal and state level. From reading Levine's book, I now understand that I am perhaps a reincarnated food reformer, because there's an old lineage of food reformers, mostly moms, who created and labored for a national school lunch program—representing one of the great driving forces on earth—a mother's need to feed her child.

According to Levine, the school lunch program is one of America's favorite welfare programs, because it seems to know how to provide reasonably healthy food and pay for it. Lunch programs vary between schools as well as between states. Nutrition standards keep altering. How lunch programs are funded shift. During all the years of the program, two important facts remain: school lunch programs are needed, and it's a struggle to provide them. Currently, there's a global movement looking at lunch programs in schools. Goodall tells a story in her *Harvest of Hope* book about how someone held up a stalk of celery to a class in the United Kingdom and not one child could identify what it was. It's slightly relieving to know that the U.S. is not alone in this problem. Many chefs are stepping in to help. There's a U.S. national farms-to-school organization. Yet, the underlying, greater challenge remains—how to economically provide fresh and whole food meals in the lunch line.

The Internet brings new leverage for lunch programs. Schools around the world are beginning to use school websites to market and inform parents regarding lunch programs and other efforts that support a healthy school and planet.

Ellen Richards, an early nutritional reformer, opened the first school lunchroom in 1898. She said poor diets and the inability to avoid bad foods weakens the moral fiber and lessens mental as well as physical efficiency.[3] The first National School Lunch Program began in the U.S. after World War II to improve the nutritional status of America's children after so many men were found unfit to serve our country. Now it compromises the health of our children. The 1920s –1950s marked a U.S. problem with underweight children. What is different and critical now is childhood obesity, juvenile diabetes, and global instability around food production and distribution.

Levine states parents can and must use their influence to protect children's health. [4] Levine's rather uninspiring closing remark on her history of school lunches is: "When it comes to children, food, and welfare, school lunch politics challenges all players—agriculture, the food-service industry, nutritionists, children's welfare advocates, and elected officials alike—to serve up balanced meals that include substantive resources along with healthy diets." [5]

My local school district, and most U.S. schools, has had to cut lunch staff, meaning there's limited workers to prepare food, thus, the need for cheap, already prepared, packaged meals. I started researching vendors for healthier school lunches. Besides the national farm-to-school organization, I found that there are several organic and conventional farming groups in California trying to reach out to schools and other organizations. I learned many orders go through an organization called Growers Collaborative, and many

---

[3] P.22, School Lunch Politics

[4] P. 228, Jane Goodall

[5] p. 191, School Lunch politics

of the separate nonprofits and farmers supply this collaborative. Under this collaborative, they offer organic and conventional, while all being locally grown. This works because a large school needs to know what they are serving a month in advance, since parents are given the menu for the month.

All-organic contacts are dependent on what the farmers can grow given the season and weather. At least conventional produce is produced locally. Still, cost, affordability, and appeal to our students are important factors. Even if we can afford pears and cucumbers and the students like them, other things must be taken into account, such as the available labor to cut this fresh produce into slices and distribute them. I hear one technique gaining ground and enjoyed by kids is food tasting. For example, zucchini is fresh out of the school garden and students see the raw zucchini, taste a stir fry or vegetable soup with zucchini and zucchini bread. This is also something our nutritional director wants to do but says she needs the kids to come out of the classroom and back to the cafeteria. I don't glorify cafeterias because combined with kids they are very loud. My sister, who is a first grade teacher, takes her students back to her classroom for lunch as a reward, because it is more pleasant to eat. Another big problem with students being in the classroom is the nutritional director is unable to monitor and assess how well the food is working.

I asked these farming organizations if they also had any leads on dairy, but no one did. It seems a realistic and broadly appealing start for change if we could get 1% hormone free milk. I went down to my local health food store and asked one of the savvy employees. She said, look up Clover.com (I remember Clover ice cream and dairy growing up. I wonder if it's originally a Wisconsin company. It used to stay on the Wisconsin license plate, "the dairy state." California now has more dairy industry and I hear it's quite politically powerful in this state. Food is really political! The dining hall at school is filled with posters of only celebrities with the milk mustache.). From the Clover website, I got a lead to a local distributor of the product. I looked at the chocolate milk. No high fructose corn syrup (HFCS). Evaporated cane juice. 30 grams of sugar per serving. Yikes. That's a lot! Not too teacher-friendly to send kids back to class after that drink.

Farm-to-school sounds great, hopeful and promising, doesn't it? Schools have budgets and need to get the school's lunch menu planned and out for the whole month. For example, we know generally that apples are available every fall, but don't always know when the apples are ready, what specific kind are available, for how long they are available, and even how much they cost, which varies week to week. Can schools become more flexible and serve seasonal, fresh local produce?

Currently, the grants for our local growers collaborative (the central connection that represents many local farms) are allocated to underfunded schools. They are mainly working on educating children from these schools, since the children are considered at a disadvantage. They do some planting with the kids, make presentations, and facilitate food tasting, but getting the farm food into the school lunch menu remains the challenge.

Deidre and I met with the nutritional director again for three hours at my home. It seemed divinely guided, our little group, Deidre a nurse and myself, a credentialed teacher. We're all parents. Our experience is pertinent to this type of situation, and Kimberly benefits from our feedback. I have understanding and respect for fellow teachers, so I come in with sensitivity to the impact of changes on teachers and school schedules. Kimberly is the best person to address with hashing out the issues at the school. She has power as the school district's nutritional director, and she is the most knowledgeable about its lunch food. In addition, another factor that brings balance to our team is that I'm a vegetarian and they're not. Deidre is very knowledgeable about food and understands what's raw and vegan, and Kimberly deals with vegan students. A team of three makes our efforts more manageable and efficient.

Getting down to the nitty-gritty of the actual food is very difficult. As I learned in *School Lunch Politics*, people can and have fought about what constitutes good lunch food all along. Some of the road blocks are:

- What kids will eat is a formidable issue.
- The lunch program is operating at loss.
- Kids like things packaged and served in familiar ways they see at the store and advertised on television.

- This school hasn't had success with serving 100% brown rice (currently, they mix white with brown rice).
- Because of public demand, manufacturers have started to address sodium, trans fat. For example, next year chicken nuggets will be breaded with whole wheat instead of white flour.
- School receives food commodities, or government subsidized foods. Outside vendors and products can't compete with these prices. The lunch program's budget can't afford peanut butter and chicken from our outside vendors.
- Kimberly won't budge with vendor on the HFCS in chocolate milk because she's been to presentations where other factors and changes have been pointed out at the same time that HFCS took off in the American diet. The chocolate milk they have has 26 grams of sugar compared to the (how much better?) evaporated cane juice at 30 grams a carton.

What's exciting is that our meetings have given the nutritional director more power and visibility. We've successfully sent the message that we aren't parents or a community that just cares about the damn test (the California school system is heavily dragged down by standardized testing of President George W. Bush's No Child Left Behind Act). Kimberly took the documents we generated and e-mailed them to her boss, the superintendent. Then the superintendent instructed that a meeting with all the school principals and the nutritional director be held as soon as possible to go over our requested changes. This means that we might not have to be bothered with gathering people for a board meeting.

The following week, twelve minutes before the expected meeting time with the nutritional director and the principals, the meeting is canceled.

While at the school, it had become clear to me what a humongous job the nutrition director has. Kids and food were everywhere, in and around the large dining hall building. Lunch period is central to a well functioning school; the overall vibe from the students was a happy one. I noticed about six different food service windows or opportunities for food and one stand. I got the impression of a food court for the middle and high school students. I've never seen so much food choice in a school, and so many more options than anything I experienced in school. Every day they get to choose from pizza, French fries a la carte, etc., in addition to the school lunch menu. The choices they have are phenomenal, and still not enough kids are buying food at school to support the program. Apart from staggering lunches, I got the strong reminder to forget about middle and high school students, and that our focus is clearly elementary kids.

Watching the elementary students get their food and eat it was interesting. The school doesn't have a dishwasher, and consequently those lunch trays that many of us grew up with the little sections for food are not used anymore, at least not in my area. Everything is served in disposable paper and plastic wrappers and containers. About one out of twelve little ones chose white milk, and the majority chose HFCS chocolate milk. There are no other desserts, such as cookies, served with the lunch. This school and many others run by what is called "offer versus serve." Students are required to take at least three food items but do not have to take everything, so many children can and do skip the fruits and vegetables. I was also struck by the two six graders standing behind the line with one other adult scooping out the rice and the like and serving. I expected high school students would be doing that to get work experience and to meet this need in the school. Also, there wasn't extra staff to stand around the line to help encourage the elementary students to make more healthy choices, like "take the celery sticks," or "those carrots look really good." The teachers have to stay with all the classroom kids who brought a lunch.

Deidre and I went into a classroom where the kids take their lunches to eat. There is a dining hall, but it is too small to house more than a couple of grade levels at the same time. We're working on bringing the students back to eat at least some of the time in the dining hall, such as harvest season. Nearly all the kids were eating outside and greatly enjoying the sunny day. Most were not sitting at the picnic tables available for them right there in the court yard outside their classroom. Instead, they merrily squatted around each other on the payment. Suddenly, we understood that changing or forcing the elementary kids to eat inside the dining hall, even with all the windows and double doors open to allow the fresh air in, is problematic.

Teachers are with their students during lunch so it is instructional time. How might the students learn good eating manners at school if daily they sit on the pavement to eat? I noticed one boy brought his lunch and he had two lollipops, one he shared with his buddy. We heard the teacher announce to the birthday boy to gather the other students around the picnic table for cupcakes. She turned to us and said, "I have two birthdays today." In general, I think people have this idea that a packed lunch is better than school lunches. I'm not sure this is the case.

It has served us well to be a small committee, Deidre, Kimberly and I, as well as to have my home, the midway point between Deidre and Kimberly, as our "operations base." The three of us were back together for another three hour meeting hammering out the issues as well as requests for Kimberly to present at her meeting with the principal, and it proved to be especially difficult to arrange *all* the school principals to gather for one half hour. We called our document, "Making Room for Health Achievers."

Kimberly eventually had her important meeting, and she promised to let us know how it went. We did not hear from her. Deidre and I were very disappointed. All this effort is on our own time. What I did learn is that I will never try to arrange a meeting again that requires all the principals from every school in the district to attend—unrealistic scheduling.

In the end, what have we accomplished? We went in after better quality and what did we gain? Did we make any improvements to actual food? Not one! Instead, we got educated. The school is serving 1%, hormone free milk. The school does serve fresh fruits and vegetables daily with their processed meats. They do keep trying to make meals fresh and from scratch but since they can't make foods like quesadillas consistently as the ones students are used to, then there is more waste and fewer lunches purchased. We learned that the government pays the school $0.26 for every meal they sell at full price. In order to keep the lunch program afloat, they have to sell lunches. The government mainly subsidizes the meats and the proteins. Consequently, no farms selling free range or grass fed chickens and eggs can compete. The only movement for growth is in grains and produce. How flexible can a school and its students be with local and seasonal foods? The best that we got were promises to increase farm-to-school interaction, organic produce, and opportunities to use less processed foods as well as to continue to maintain the whole foods they currently offer. What we accomplished off the page was the need and desire for more information and marketing of the lunch program on the school website. For example, the school did remove all sodas from the campus vending machines two years ago. We encouraged the school to put more information about the lunch program on the website besides just the monthly menu, and that idea was readily accepted. Parents will be able to be better informed in the new school year regarding lunch time.

Instead what happened on our mission, much like this book, is that we got at the how. We got at the issues and goals of *how we feed our children.*

Deidre and I decided to go before the school board. I asked myself, what am I really trying to do? I know the superintendent. "The Sup" has many serious issues: deciding on how many teachers she has to authorize to be laid off or not, overseeing an impossible budget, and this lunch food problem has been a struggle since its inception. Still, this is very important. I don't want to give up. I needed to prepare myself to answer the board's unspoken question: "Who are you people and why are you here bothering us?"

I had to submit a request to get on the agenda, and I received a surprising call from the Sup. She was very pleasant on the phone. I brought up one possible solution for extra help, which is to reinstate some kind of community service requirement at the high school level. She said she did not want community service because of the number of students who were "couch surfing." I told her, "I understand. Although many students are very capable of and would benefit from community service hours, there is a percentage that would not graduate with such a requirement." I did not elaborate that I had experience with helping students behind on credits make them up by doing work on campus during school hours.

Deidre and I were happy that another local father, Tim, showed up for the board meeting. It took me a day to recover from my inadequacy to present effectively and to solidify any real plans.

Deidre did a better job than myself in presenting. What happened was what I was afraid was going happen: after I asked for approval to update the school website more on its garden and more about its school-to-farm activities, the school board's response was simply, "Okay." There was no discussion, clarification, or commitment to who would be responsible and what updating the website would entail. *One* sentence could be added and the school could claim, "Yes, we updated the website."

I briefly closed my eyes hoping for some divine guidance. I was concerned about the unsustainable number of voluntary hours this effort was requiring of me, but wanting progress. A general conflict is that the people who *are* interested in better school lunches are parents who are already inundated with enough activities. How can any work get done when allocating precious free time is nearly impossible? The school is under so much pressure with basic operation and budget cuts. There's not enough staff, money, or standards to support this important effort.

I found myself struggling with the clarity and language to address the problems. I said sincerely, "We've been putting forth a lot of effort here, and we're not really getting anywhere." The Sup offered, "That's not true. At the last meeting we decided to increase the lunch fee to $3.00." She then added that it was not appropriate to have brought this issue before the board. Knowing full well that we made every effort not to have had to come to this meeting and burden the superintendent with these issues, I asked, "Who should we work with then?" A board member suggested the site council. Later, when I contacted the site council lead, she emailed me back to say that she was not the appropriate person to take this matter up with.

The Board of Trustee's Kip spoke up. "Sue, I would be willing to help you with your efforts with the lunch program. It is in our interest that the lunch program does better. I would think there would be a lot of parents interested in organics in this community."

I thanked him, the Sup, and the rest of the board for their time. I felt some relief and hope from Trustee's' interjection. Tim, Deidre, and I left feeling encouraged that we had the support of one board member.

The next day, I lay on the lounge chair in my back yard under the soft sunlight, surrounded by my pink, white, peach and yellow rose bushes and seriously questioned myself for yesterday's duress. As I relaxed, I promised myself never to go in front of the school board again. Searching for some relief, I recalled Rabbi Hillel's famous quote: "If I am not for myself, then who will be for me? And if I am only for myself, what am I? And if not now, when?" I thought indignantly, "What good are those chicken nuggets in the school lunch when they come via force fed chickens, living in miserable conditions, injected with antibiotics, and who knows what kind of slaughtering conditions? Do we want our kids to have that cheap, fatty meat, and when it comes at such expense?" I cheered myself up by recalling our progress. We've now gotten the attention of *all* the school district's leaders. Many organizations are aware of this effort in the valley now, too. The Sup did say she would see to it that the website got updated regarding these programs: gardens, lunch, and the school's farm partnership. It was a grand moment when one of the board members, the trustee, volunteered to support our efforts. I smiled. We've got a board member on our side.

At the very least, updating the school website on these programs can provide all the information that Kimberly, Deidre, and I have work so hard to find out. In this way, we, the school and the nutrition director do not have to be questioned with the same stuff again and again by the next called-to-action parents who come along. We can say, "Have you looked at the school website?" We will give the school some time next fall to get the website updates done, which seemed reasonable to me at the time. I concluded that we would contact the nutritional director mid-October to see how it's going.

Because I was not able to gather any solid accountability at the school board meeting, a whole year later, there were no changes or updates to the school website. Because of my own responsibilities and time constraints, I was reluctant to re-involve myself, but there was a lot of work that needed to be done that hadn't gotten in a whole year. I jumped through hoops with different principals to get information I needed: about the lunch program, school gardens, farm-to-school activities on the district websites. I welcomed the greater impact of working at the district level but did not take pleasure in the complications and gridlock. It is much easier working for change at only one school as opposed to a whole district.

A month later after the board meeting and at the school district's swimming pool one day, I ran into Mary, the garden instructor. (The school mainly uses its small garden for science lessons. It's called the Life Lab.) She told me about an open house at a nearby farm, Shumei, the farm-to-school program. Interesting. We haven't heard about Shumei at all except by this serendipitous moment.

Deidre and I went to the Shumei open house. I wasn't too excited about going to a farm on a hot Sunday like this one, but boy were we glad we went! Shumei represents an international natural growing foods community and the twenty-three acres farm in Bonny Doon is owned by all its members. The Japanese community came out for the event so it was well attended. The food, the Taiko drummers, and more, were outlandishly remarkable.

At the event, I tracked down our busy contact person. After introducing myself, she said excitedly, "I want to work with you guys! We will match any price you're paying!" Maybe Kimberly can plan the monthly lunch menu by putting, for example, "apple and celery sticks or other fresh, locally grown, seasonal, organic produce." This could turn lunch sales around completely!

An online article reports that lunch lines weren't moving fast enough for a Boulder Valley, Colorado school district and, consequently, kids barely had enough time to sit and eat before the lunch period was over. [6] So, when we're having problems just trying to get kids to buy lunch here, lunch time crunch is a problem elsewhere.

October came around and soon enough, more volunteers were crawling out of the woodworks. Now it seems that the nation, in general, has a general consciousness about the obesity epidemic, school lunches, and buying local. Our next meeting was attended by

---

[6]

http://www.time.com/time/business/article/0,8599,1665119,00.html

---

28

a number of prominent school administrators, garden people, and parents. In closing the meeting, we did discuss a name separate from the school's wellness policy. We wanted to come up with something that included our school district name, nutrition requirements and had a fun or clever acronym, but people were stumped along with me. We finally came up with SLV LOCALS (San Lorenzo Valley Local Organic Children's Advocates for Lunches in Schools), and a yet another yahoo group was born.

Linda, from Shumei, gave me a video to watch called "Hidden Dangers in Kid's Meals," which is about how corporate influence and government collusion work in tandem to cover up serious health dangers in food. In it was the same school shown in the film, "Super Size Me." I followed up and discovered that the two people who were supporting the whole effort retired, and the people on the other end of the line and the website had no further leads.

I understand why that video ended in a dead end. Without Deidre cheering me on and others showing up to support us, it would be too discouraging. The disheartening part still is that the nutritional director never responds to email, and a lot of work and progress gets done via email. She rarely calls me back, and I don't call that often. When I simply must have some information from her, I call her after she hasn't called me and we talk and I understand once again that so much of this is new territory for her and above and beyond an already demanding job. Providing healthy lunches in public schools is a justice issue. It's not right that kids in private schools get quality lunches and all the other kids don't. One parenting book sums the issue up nicely:

"Let's look at a short list of things that children are fully entitled to: respectful treatment, **healthful food**, shelter from the weather, practical and comfortable clothing, yearly checkups at the pediatrician and the dentist, and a good education. Everything else is a privilege."[7]

One of the next efforts came with completing a Hidden Valley Ranch grant online application. Hidden Valley Ranch found in two Northern California studies that many children will eat more fresh

---

[7] The Blessing of a Skinned Knee," Wendy Mogel, Ph.D.

vegetables if they have ranch dressing for dip. Consequently, Hidden Valley Ranch was offering ten $15,000 grants to schools with a fresh veggies plan. I couldn't imagine we were going to have that much competition for the grant because answering all the questions felt like writing a thesis. Kimberly, Deidre, and I met late into the evening to finish up our application.

When the February Hidden Valley Ranch winner announcement time arrived, we found out we didn't win. I realized then that no one is going to come save us. Our community doesn't have money, but we don't qualify as desperate enough to be gifted any outside help.

At yet another meeting, we got lucky. A mature, local, nutritional chef, Kathy, attended our meeting. At this same meeting, Kimberly agreed to try one-day-a-week natural foods day. The general feeling at the meeting was, "I hope it works."

The following week, Chef Kathy and I met one on one to generate some mainly vegetarian entree and recipe ideas to offer the lunch program for the last six Natural Foods Wednesdays, and Kathy took it upon herself to scale the recipes. I've learned along the way that Kimberly's strongest skills are managing people and numbers to run a large school dining hall, but definitely not large-scale cooking.

Kimberly, Chef Kathy, and I met again to finalize some ideas. We talked over the details of doing bean enchiladas. Chef Kathy said, "Easy! You lay down a layer of your tortilla, the rice, the beans, the cheese, the sauce, and another layer of tortilla." They figure out how many servings they can get out of the industrial pans. Kimberly says they can't do it. "I don't have enough time or staff to get the job done." Because of the union, we can't use any volunteers either—not that we could get any. I said, "Okay, simply beans and rice." We all agreed. Kimberly could do it. We determined two other entrees: polenta pizza and something else. If any of them worked, Kimberly and Kathy could repeat them on another Wednesday.

Then, the first day of the last six Wednesdays of the school year arrived—the school's first Natural Foods Wednesday. Three hundred, and hopefully fifty new families, will eat black beans and rice (half white, half brown) and organic salad from the local Shumei Farm.

I created and sent fliers to be put up in the lunch line about black beans along with some popular cartoon characters to get the kids who don't eat beans to buy into the whole food idea.

What's Nifty, Nice, New, and Nutritional in the Lunch Line?

Natural Foods Wednesday!

New lunch menus made from scratch with whole foods and local organic vegetables. Lunch price is the same: $3.00.

When? May 6th – June 10th

(Last Six Wednesdays of the School Year)

Who?

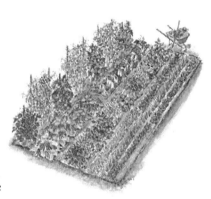

San Lorenzo Valley Nutrition Services with Shumei Natural Agriculture farm supplying fresh, locally grown, organic salads.

Enjoy and make the lunch program stronger by supporting these special end-of-the-year meals!

Even after Linda from Shumei gave a brochure to be put in all the teacher's mailboxes, not one class scheduled a spring field trip. When Linda told me that, I asked if she would host one for preschoolers and she agreed. I organized with seven mom friends and their kids and a few younger siblings to go. A month later we went. We looked for redwood tree seeds, which are about the size of one grain of brown rice—remarkable for the tallest tree on the planet. We learned a little about Ohlone Indians who once lived on the land, had salad from the garden, and the children planted zucchini and sunflowers seeds.

On the way out, we got to stop by and see the greenhouse with the lettuce growing for the children at our two elementary schools. Upon seeing it my mom friend, Paula, said "This is what you guys have done? I feel like crying."

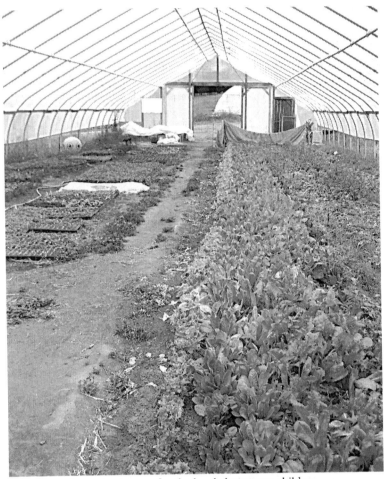

Shumei growing lettuce for the local elementary children.

Shumei doesn't use any toxic fertilizers (not even animal manure). Being on it felt safe and sacred. My friend with a toddler wasn't worried about any dirt her daughter was getting into. On the contrary, she was hoping that being on the farm was building her immunity. And we all got to feel good that we were able to provide the finest kind of environment for our children—nourishing and natural.

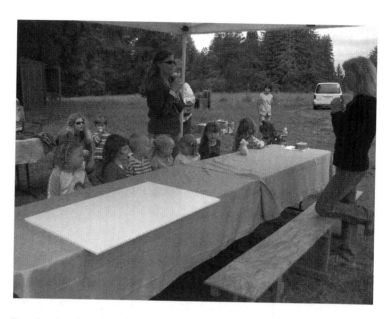

Preschoolers learning about natural agriculture at Shumei, 2009.

The week before, a story about the Natural Foods Wednesday ran in our local weekly paper. I had contacted a journalist who agreed to do one. I not only wanted more energy moving towards the efforts and parent awareness, I needed the school lunch program to follow through. The obstacles are never ending, and public attention is what Kimberly needed to work through to something new and better.

Kids love lunch time. Lunch period has tremendous potential for learning, health and fun. I wish the effort could be easier, but I believe we are backing our way out of a bad situation into a brighter future.

After the first Natural Foods Wednesday, Kimberly, Chef Kathy, farm managers, and I met. Kimberly said it went well. The first thing she showed us was her numbers. Compared to the previous Wednesday, she sold 40 more lunches, so the Natural Foods Wednesday was having a positive effect. We implored her about the food. She said, "The beans and rice looked and tasted really good. On their way back to eat their lunch, some of the kids stopped to throw out their salad or the entre directly. But the salad was so beautiful with the variety of green lettuces with the snow peas, and accents of radishes were great." Given the Japanese reputation for floral arrangement, its meticulousness and elegance, I was sure that the salad was indeed presented artfully.

I asked about any responses from the article in the paper. Kimberly said, "My staff was happy and excited about it, but I did not receive one comment from the principal or other teachers. However, I am excited that the garden teacher came down and offered to bring in her class before Natural Foods Wednesday next week to help prep the lunch—tear up the lettuce for the salad." Kimberly said excitedly, "It is what I've wanted for so long."

Then the farm manager said he just got two new interns in and asked if he could bring them to work at the school as part of their training. Kimberly said yes. I felt happy to see the mutually benefiting relationship happening. All in all, everyone was delighted about our progress.

We ended with the fact that we have a nearby farmers market on Tuesdays that runs from spring to fall, but how do we regularly get someone to pick up at 6:30 in the evening to glean what was left and then get to the school when nobody is there? There's no budget, programs, or high-level support for such efforts. I was surprised and pleased to hear Kimberly say: "I will go to the market myself and pick it up, if that's what it takes."

Deidre called the next day to see if I was going to the nearby farmers market to work on the gleaning effort and to try to connect with a particular farm, "Happy Boy Farm." I responded dismally that I couldn't keep giving this much time or effort, but in the end, I caved, and said, "Oh, all right." Well, I found them and got an immediate bright response. I thought about how often people do want to help the schools, children, and be involved, but it requires people working together, sacrificing, giving and figuring out how to make it work. The young and welcoming tattooed, nose pierced, and blue-haired woman working for Happy Boy Farm replied quickly, "The person needs to be here at 6:30 to pick up with their own boxes. We already work an eleven hour day so we can't be responsible for getting it to the school afterwards, but we do want our leftover fresh, organic lettuce and other produce like melons to go to the school." I called Kimberly and left a message with the woman's contact information.

I was shocked to hear Kimberly's message on my answering machine when I got home later that evening. She had picked up Happy Boy's leftover produce. Said it was beautiful and that she will have enough tomorrow for even the high school salad bar.

On the second year now, the gleaning efforts continue. Kimberly continues to pick up on Tuesday evenings when the market is open as there's no additional staff or hours to support that pick up. Another new Saturday farmers market opened up, and SLVLOCALS continues to organize and glean when we can from this market. We successfully arranged with a local convention center to store the produce in its refrigeration until Monday morning when Kimberly can pick it up before school. Our goal is to bring in more volunteers to help with the pick up to consistently be at the markets for gleaning.

I've seen my chiropractor's family attend the farmers market regularly. I worked to get her on board, and her receptionist, a high school mom with two boys, quipped, "Yeah, instead of throwing it away at the farmers market, the kids can throw it away at school." I replied with a smile, "We're working on that part, too!"

Sugarless Strategies

Shortly after my daughter turned three and a half, I enrolled her in a dance class. I had a beautiful hour of spring time all to myself, and then went to pick up Savanah. She had a large plastic egg with two colorfully wrapped treats inside fascinating her. As I put her in the car I couldn't think of a clever way of getting the goods from her. She opened the small lollipop and instinctively popped it in her mouth. Smiling from ear to ear and in an incredulous way she exclaimed, "Momma, what is this?" I told the truth with no enthusiasm: "It's candy."

Our children now consume unprecedented levels of processed sugar. Hidden sugar in foods along with the obvious sweets in children's diets is sabotaging their health. Children do have a formidable sweet tooth. Mother's milk is sweet. Sugar would hardly be an issue if children ate sweets here and there, but hardly a week, neigh a day, can go by without some outing, holiday, birthday party, parents or friends giving our kids treats. Sugar is a source of unease for me, fellow parents, and an enormous problem for Americans.

One of the many difficulties with refined white sugar is that it is highly concentrated and void of any nutritional value. It is an artificial, manmade substance that is a foreign invader to the body. As children quickly become accustomed to the intense sweet taste of this non-natural sugar, the less they are able to enjoy the ordinary sweetness found in whole foods like vegetables. Despite my understanding of refined sugar and all its demises to our health, I can't keep my daughter away from it. At best, I try to set limits and continue to be vigilant about its ubiquitous presence.

While living in Dallas many years ago, I stumbled upon a health group that focused on abstaining from all white flour and sugar. *What an interesting focus*, I thought. I liked what I heard, and the next day I went cold turkey on all white flour and sugar products. I went through withdrawal. It was like quitting an addiction. I had a wretched, hang over-like headache. I was tired and felt discouraged.

I walked around in a daze. On day three, I found myself weeping off and on. I couldn't believe how difficult it was. And then on day four, I felt great. My mind felt clearer than it had for a very long time.

From that first day, I was able to maintain and stop eating any refined white flour or sugar for close to a year straight.

This marvelous experience stays with me. To this day, this experience proves to me that refined sugar is a drug. It dulls the mind. I felt and saw myself drift out of foggy, illusive dream. My mind started to think and run faster. During my first months of abstinence, I witnessed the explosion of the Internet. While so many of us in my generation were struggling to learn new computer and software programs, I felt I had an advantage over my coworkers with my clearer, quicker-thinking mind. Mostly, I just enjoyed feeling physically better. Unfortunately, I haven't been able to consistently maintain my liberty from refined white flour and sugar. It's not an easy thing for most of us to do, and I find it even more difficult to stay off of refined flour and sugar during these child-rearing years.

I took my daughter to her first day of a morning summer soccer camp. Once again, I picked her up from a *sports program*, and she was wearing a candy bracelet as part of her reward for attending the camp. It seems everyone wants the kids to be happy in *their* program, and candy works every time. My neighbor took her daughter to the same camp and her older son to a different soccer camp the same week and she said, "When I picked up Aiden just before lunch, the kids there were all eating an ice cream sandwich."

Part of me wants to be the good guy, too, the one who gets to pass out the treats. It's fun. Kids *love* the taste and delight in the many colorful shapes, ingredients, and wrappers. Everyone enjoys seeing happy children, and it's not pleasant being with an unhappy one. I see that junk food and sweets flood our child's daily life. I've got to do my best to make the food at home as whole and fresh as possible, not that that's easy, but it sure only goes downhill outside the home.

On the topic of sugar, I found helpful Ann Louise Gittleman's *Get the Sugar Out: 501 Simple Ways to Cut the Sugar Out of Any Diet*. This book addresses the multifaceted subject of sugar. Gittleman names and explains the sweet differences between nearly all the natural, refined and artificial sugars, as well as the new players in the market, like the sugar alcohols. It was even more enlightening during my second read of it. Her book rouses my effort to continue reading the labels. She writes: "There's just no way around it. If you're going to buy packaged foods, you have to pay attention to what's in them. Three-quarters of the sugars Americans ingest are hidden in processed foods."[1] Three-quarters of the sugar our children ingest isn't even the obvious: cookies, ice cream and candy? What does Gittleman mean by "hidden sugars"?

Hidden Sugars

When Savanah was four, I started looking at children's multivitamins. I was flabbergasted when the salesclerk at my health food store offered me trial tastings, a delightful tasting, sugar-coated gum drop and said this was a children's multivitamin. "Sticky candy injected with nutrients," she explained. "Gosh, my child might beg and sneak multivitamins if I brought something like that home," I said, "Do you have any whole foods multivitamins without sugar, maybe just flavored would be okay?" She said, "Nope, none exist [yet]." Later, I ask the same soccer mom neighbor about vitamins and she said, "I use the liquid form and the kids take it no problem but don't beg for it."

One day I sat down for lunch outside our local health food store with another mom. We looked at the sugar content of the yogurt we both just bought for our kids. It was the first time I bought yogurt for Savanah and was looking for some fast food because she didn't want a piece of fruit. The mom and I both had a different yogurt and each one had about 26 grams of sugar. Four grams equal one teaspoon of white sugar. So that means these cute, easy to grab, feed your kid, no brainer, "healthy," little colorful containers of yogurt have the equivalent of almost *seven* teaspoons of sugar. I'm hoping some of it is the milk sugar, the lactose, and the rest is sucrose or fructose. It still adds up to sugar. (Later I checked out a similar size plain yogurt. It has 10 grams of lactose sugar.) After the

---

[1] Page 71, Ann Louise Gittleman's Get the Sugar Out: 501 Simple Ways to Cut the Sugar Out of Any Diet

snack, my friend's two year old son acted loopy and was hanging upside down from the bench and wiggling and grinning. Maybe it was just little boy stuff, but I got the feeling he was having a sugar rush.

The next week when I found some free time, I returned to the health store with a paper and pen and read yogurt labels from two cooler doors and twelve shelves of yogurt. Every purchase is a vote and responsibility, but how many mothers with two little ones in tow can make an informed choice? For a half hour, I studied many of the mostly organic yogurts and couldn't even get to all the brands. California is the largest producer of dairy foods in the U.S. Why would I buy these yogurts in the case from Canada or from the east coast when I live in California? One reason many of us try to shop at health foods stores is we want them to help us by selling products that have a higher standard of health for people and the planet, and here I am talking about the yogurt at a health food store. I know they're trying to do everything they can to keep the customers happy with what sells. It's overwhelming just to figure out what yogurt to buy our child. Is it any wonder many of us just throw in the towel and buy what's on sale? We shouldn't have to, nor do we have time to sit around and study labels all the time. Who wants to spend their life doing that?

I found that the single serving yogurts with 26-32 grams of sugar mark the high end of hidden sugar in yogurt. I figure one goal is to try to buy yogurt with less than 26 grams of sugar (that a child likes— which is the challenge once they've had "the good stuff"), is made locally (roughly within a 150 mile radius), and has live and active cultures added after pasteurizing.

The next day I stopped by a commercial grocery store to buy spaghetti sauce—déjà vu— shelves and shelves of spaghetti sauce. I didn't have time for this. I grabbed something organic. I got home and read the label. Second ingredient: sugar. Consumers are being misled by the upstaging of the term "organic" on labels.

Not only are consumers misled by false advertising and labeling, but also inadvertently by health gurus who advocate nutritious ingredients in recipes that commonly use brown sugar as an alternative. In *Hypoglycemia: The Classic Healthcare Handbook*, Saunders also once thought brown sugar was a nutritional alternative to white sugar until she actually visited several sugar refineries in Hawaii and California.[2] "Light brown [sugar] is 88 percent white sugar; dark brown is 87 percent, and kleenraw is 95 percent. [White sugar] is refined to the point of foodlessness, containing neither vitamins nor minerals, and is a definite human health hazard." Saunders tells a gripping story of a mother and daughter's devastation with sugar in chapter one of *Hypoglycemia*. She lost her daughter as a young adult, and she points to sugar as a major contributor. This book had me seriously reflecting on the level and role of sugar in student behavior problems in school and violence in society in general.

HFCS

High Fructose Corn Syrup (HFCS) is very unhealthy, and I'm happy that people are increasingly becoming more aware of this. I am glad I was able to break the menacing grips of drinking canned soda myself many years ago, as these products are one of the biggest offenders. I am always disheartened when I see children drinking sodas, but if the parents drink soda, which many of us do, then it's quite difficult to keep soda away from kids.

Both Gittleman and Barbara Kingsolver in her book, *Animal, Vegetable, Miracle*, talk about the evils of this particular processed sugar. Kingsolver describes the environmental devastation from corn production. Gittleman addresses HFCS on the first page of her book:

"HFCS is perhaps the most insidious of all sugar substitutes.[3] By replacing sugar with HFCS, you can override your body's natural ability to feel full, so you eat more. Without this type of signal you don't know when to stop eating. Now that is downright scary."[4]

I talked with a mom friend about HFCS. She said her son was having the worst gas ever and for the family's sake, they needed to find out what he was eating at school to cause this unlivable situation. Her son is slightly lactose intolerant and she found out he

---

2 Page 140, *Hypoglycemia: The Classic Healthcare Handbook*

3 Page 1, Ann Louise Gittleman's *Get the Sugar Out: 501 Simple Ways to Cut the Sugar Out of Any Diet*

4 Page 7 Gittleman

was having the school's chocolate milk. She read the label and the second ingredient in the chocolate milk was HFCS.

One challenge I found in trying to get HFCS out of the lunch program is that alternative chocolate milk made with evaporated cane sugar had more sugar grams then the current HFCS brand they used. It's also amazing to me that getting chocolate milk out of the school lunch program is too big of an issue for me to tackle. One online mom wrote that chocolate milk was the only way to get her child to drink milk, so she and others did not seem interested in seeing it disappear from the school lunch menu. Drinking milk is a big part of the conventional American diet.

When HFCS became common place in the late 1970s, obesity levels began to soar, and corn syrup has been directly linked to the rising levels of obesity.[5] Some people dispute this saying there were other factors and changes occurring at the same time. HFCS is a highly processed, cheap, super-sweet version of white table sugar and it is found in just about every food in our supermarkets, including baby formulas. Corn is the number one crop grown in the U.S., and it is subsidized by the government. Industrialized corn farmers sell the cheap corn as feed for the meat production. No longer do our animals graze on grass like they used to not so long ago. The corn diet has changed the meat quality and made it, for one, higher in saturated fat. Corn farmers rely heavily on agrochemicals, which cause enormous damage to the environment. Vast amounts of tropical rain forests have been destroyed to grow corn to feed cattle for our heavy meat consumption. HFCS is one ingredient I've gotten serious about.

Chocolate and sugar have a successful marriage, and chocolate is a main character in our culture. Savanah does not like chocolate. Whenever she says she doesn't want the chocolate being offered, stops people dead in their tracks. The multitude of us chocolate lovers is mystified; we can't wrap our brain around not liking chocolate. I'm having fun just writing about chocolate. I've asked Savanah about what she is going to say at school when other children scream: "What! You don't like chocolate?" We were at a birthday party and a very fit and health-conscious mother made a

---

[5] Page 7?? Gittleman, Get the sugar out

game of hiding gummy worms under a pile of whip cream sprinkled with chocolate. The kids couldn't use their hands and had to get to the candy using their mouth only. When I asked her to make one without chocolate for Savanah she smiled and said, "She'll grow out of it." Recently after Savanah finished two weeks of swimming lessons, the kids were offered small chocolate bars. Savanah was disappointed. Her chocolate-loving swim pal beamed in Savanah's face while she smacked on her chocolate reward and with a wide smile said, "Yummm!" Savanah scowled back. I took Savanah to a raw food chocolate presentation by David Wolfe when she was about two or three years old, fed her some chocolate there, and she's hated the stuff ever since. I don't keep chocolate handy for myself, so that also has a lot of influence on Savanah's disinterest.

I've concluded that one thing we can do is continue to educate ourselves about the kinds of foods we're purchasing, and be more vigilant about the disguised sugary foods and products like the spaghetti sauce with its hidden sugar. Since time is forever a challenge, I often talk with fellow friends about various products we use. Everywhere I find that parents are interested in discussions on healthier products, shopping tips, money saving and more local or ethical companies.

There are products nearly impossible to buy without some sugar, like most cereals. It's common knowledge now that the first ingredients make up the bulk of a product. There's a rule of five used by many, which is to look for the sugar *after* the first five ingredients.

Another thing I do is not keep white sugar in our house. When I was a kid, we regularly had a sugar bowl filled with white, refined sugar (sucrose) on the breakfast table that we used to pour liberally on our breakfast cereal and oatmeal, which sounds outlandish today. Some sweet substitutes I use are Stevia, agave, honey, Xylitol, and fruit juice.

Everyday's a Party

Holidays give structure, meaning, and delight to our children. I enjoy holidays now more than I did as a child, because I am now raising one of my own and see how much more special it is for her. Children need variety. They like drama and excitement with food;

they love the thrill and anticipation. Food is an important part of many holidays. Every celebration I consider the food traditions I am going to do or not do and how to create my own. It's a challenge.

For example, we don't have a big turkey at Thanksgivings, and I want to avoid all refined sugar, so I consider what honors my ideas about nourishing food and what's going to delight my child. At the same time, there's this general current or justification we have in this culture: "Hey, relax a little, it's Halloween (Christmas, Aiden's birthday, Valentine's Day, Fourth of July parade, summer vacation, Grandma's visiting, Grandma's not visiting, it's the weekend)—live a little!" And here we have a health and sugar expert, Gittleman, who says that our *number one priority* is to get all the refined white sugar out of the diet because it's been implicated in some sixty different diseases.[6] She says, we need to avoid refined sugar at all costs.[7] What a rock and a hard place for parents. I'm a community person. I'm out living life with my daughter. Everywhere we go it's a dietary party. I know that sugar is really bad for Savanah and all the children, but we're entrenched in it.

Valentine's Day. Some of my friends go to a religious based preschool and some American holidays aren't celebrated like Halloween and Valentines Day because they're considered pagan holidays. I can see this as a sweet advantage. When Savanah was four and in preschool for the first time, Valentine's Day took me a bit by surprise. I do enjoy the arts and crafts that come with the holidays as they provide ideas and opportunities for writing, cutting, gluing—fine motor, prewriting skills, and the focus of completing projects. I learned that the other children had each brought little candies and stuff. I also noticed out and about how the commercialization and celebrating of this holiday keeps getting bigger and bigger every year like Halloween—that's the way it is in the states. I took Savanah out and she bought each girl a new, character toothbrush like Dora the Explorer. These preschool kids loved their new toothbrushes. I figure it was 40 or whatever less grams of sugar. To not be wasteful, I like the pencils and other little

---

[6] Page 34 Gittleman

[7] Page 28 Gittleman

practical gifts as well. Savanah ended up having two candies, and I was glad that she did not go to a large preschool.

Not only is the beware of hidden sugars strategy important, here's where feeding vegetables for breakfast strategy that I talk about later in this book works, if and when we can pull it off. Savanah had eaten celery sticks and other raw vegetables Valentine's Day morning, and so I was less disconcerted by the day's candies, and glad she didn't start out with hot chocolate and a donut, another common breakfast, especially during the winters.

As far as more ideas for Valentines Day, we wrote Daddy a love poem, which took much more thought and time than I expected. Poems appear easy. My girl friend's husband gave flowers to her and to each of their little girls. Another family with older kids gave each other love coupons, like to get out of a chore, or for a new book. I was dispirited to hear my friend, who is health conscious and struggles terribly with her teenage daughter's mood swings, gave her daughter a heart box of chocolates. This is one reason I keep talking about health and food ideas with friends. We forget! We are unintentionally harming our children with sugar.

Halloween. Halloween is a favorite holiday for kids and many parents. It's a sweet holiday that's tough to get around. When my daughter was two, I took her out with me on errands that day. Had I recalled how nuts people have become over this holiday I would have planned not to go out that day at all, as she was terrified by the people in costume at nine a.m. in the morning! The bride of Frankenstein and the Samoa wrestler stand out in my memory. She had to talk about it for months afterwards to work through her trauma.

Parents come up with clever stuff for dealing with the candy. I know many parents who let their kids trick or treat and then turn their candy bag over in exchange for a toy or special outing and it works! There's a fairy story available online called, "The Sugar Sprites," and it's about gathering candy to leave for the fairies to eat during the winter. I know one parent who had a grand time trick or treating with her three year olds who loved the story and successfully avoided the junk. Sometimes I run out of cleverness. I understand why so many parents just give up on abstaining from the candy and junk food. They get tired of what feels like a losing battle.

It's Halloween again. This year I bought chocolate mini candy bars, gum, and Play-Doh. I asked the kid who came dressed as a garbage can (the lid was the hat and he cut leg holes into the large Rubbermaid) if he wanted Play Doh or candy. "Candy!" he said without hesitation. The rest of the night I was only able to give the Play Doh to the clueless, cute three year olds at the door. The gum went well even though chewing gum isn't the most princess-like behavior.

I tried countless so-called healthy recipes with alternative ingredients that fail with kids. I tried at least a dozen raw recipes from *Eating Without Heating*, which was written by teenagers and very colorful. Everyone was awash!

Thanksgiving. Thanksgiving has been a completely new challenge for me. I grew up with much of the traditional fare: turkey, stuffing, cranberry sauce, and pumpkin pie. At four, my daughter had her first taste of pumpkin pie made with love by our friend, the kind that can't go wrong with kids: graham cracker crust made with half a cup of white sugar. She came home and we made my healthier version of pumpkin pie made without any crust at all. The next morning she woke up begging for pumpkin pie. I gave her a slice of our pie and after her first taste, she wailed in despair, "Nooo!" I laugh now but at the time I felt awful!

Fourth of July. When Savanah was a toddler we went to a winter holiday parade, and all the candy throwing got past her. I didn't take her to another parade for many years even though there are many annual ones close to home. When Savanah was five and half, I took her to a Fourth of July parade, and broke the news about what happens at parades and how candy gets thrown. She couldn't wait to go this parade. We sat at the beginning of the parade where it wasn't too crowded, and we were showered with candy. I have to say it is gobs of fun to see candy flying all over the place. I got into the whole thing. "Run Savanah! Over there! There's more! Get it! Oh, get that one!" We left with at least one hundred pieces of candy. Now what? I didn't think this thing through. I couldnn't let her eat all that candy, even if I doled it out a few pieces at a time. I didn't want it in the house. I didn't want her begging and sneaking for candy. She got to eat some of the candy. I did a special outing trade with her, and when we went to the fireworks later on, I threw the rest of it in a garbage can as she watched. She'll probably remember that trash can by the tennis courts for the rest of her life: "That's the garbage can where my mom threw my Fourth of July candy away."

Birthdays. What's a child's birthday party without a birthday cake? I do think we can limit our birthday parties to just that—a piece of cake or cupcake. I gave my daughter her first birthday party at the age of four. She went to a birthday party the weekend before where she had a "real" white sugar and flour, frosted princess cake. I used to know how to make chocolate mousse and cheesecakes. In fact, I worked as a part-time baker while in graduate school. For my daughter's fourth birthday, I didn't even make her a homemade birthday cake, which I wanted to, but I was afraid after my pumpkin pie fiasco at Thanksgiving.

I received the online photos of a birthday party we missed. I saw another gigantic piñata filled with candy. Piñatas are another sugar feast ritual that's become standard, which sometimes sends kids home with a Halloween-like bag of candy. A few older moms one day who have "been there, done that," all laughed when I exclaimed, "I hate birthdays and holidays! All the candy and sugar!" I know one mom who just plain didn't take her kids to birthday parties for the first seven or so years of their lives. She had two boys close in age who were play mates for each other. Having just given my first child's birthday party, I completely understand the need to make it special. Since Savanah doesn't have any siblings, she needs outside friends and activities. Some parents are able to offer parties at skating rinks or rock climbing gyms, which give the kids great exercise while having fun.

After reading a book that had a blueberry pie in it, I mentioned to Savanah how much I loved my grandmother's blueberry pie when I was a young girl. Blueberries are plentiful and common in the summers in Wisconsin and Michigan where I was raised, while blackberries are the thing along California's central coast. After reading that book, Savanah often asked for blueberry pie.

My friend, Jennifer, and our daughters and I went blackberry picking one day for the purpose of gathering enough berries to make a pie. Blackberries are delicate and usually not ripe, thus sour, in the stores so I hardly ever buy them; not to mention, they are expensive. We picked all our blackberries for free, which made it even more fun. The girls delighted in picking hand to mouth while the moms filled the buckets. As we picked, I thought about how the blackberry pie makes for a fun and special connection with the season.

Because Miss Health Kick me got rid of most of my baking paraphernalia, the next day Savanah and I went over to Jennifer's to make the blackberry pie. The pie turned out beautifully and as I ate my piece, I could not imagine anything that tasted better than that homemade blackberry pie. Savanah, being the delicate eater that she is, dipped her fork into the dripping, warm-cooked blackberry and took a teeny tiny taste. She put her fork down in disappointment and quietly said, "I don't like it." "All the more for the rest of us," I responded.

For Savanah's fifth birthday, I tried a "promised to be amazing" Silken tofu frosting recipe. Savanah took one taste: "Yuck! Mommy, you better buy a cake!" As a last minute surrender, I bought a Hello Kitty cake with hyper-activity causing, trans-fat frosting. Of course, the kids loved it. And it was struggle for me not to cave in to Savanah's begging for a piñata. Filling up a piñata with cheap little toys instead of candy also isn't very green and not a great alternative to the piñatas dilemma.

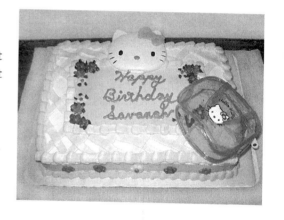

Once I queried one of my parent online groups about birthday treats at school as one way of cutting back and controlling the amount of unnatural sugar in children's diet and helping with their overall health. I wrote: "I would like to hear what other parents think about bringing birthday treats to school. Did a SLV school lunch observation today. What a production feeding all those kids!

While there, I heard one teacher announce to the other students to gather around the table for the cupcakes. Then commented to me, 'I have two birthdays today.'"

I continued with my post. "Since we lose significant control over what our kids actually eat when they begin school and much more so as they get older, the birthday party treats might be something to consider. My sister-in-law told me about her boys in a CastroValley, CA Elementary School. The school sent out notices letting parents knows that birthday cupcakes and candies were no longer going to be accepted during the school day. The notice stated carrot sticks, fruit, and raisins were okay, and stated that they could deliver any sweets they liked after school.

Everyone wins with this situation. Parents don't have the pressure of having to keep up with the other parents. A child doesn't have to feel bad for not being able to bring treats on their birthday. It's a great way to honor, show respect, and care for the teachers because many children have negative reactions to sugar and chocolate and, consequently, this policy saves the teachers from distracting behaviors in the classroom. Finally, the kids benefit from less junk food at school. Maybe this is just a 'whatever' topic? Let parents do whatever they want. If they want to send their child to school on his or her birthday with a three-layer chocolate cake, let 'em! Thanks for any comments."

I was surprised that the responses added up to: "Bringing treats for a birthday is fine; it means a lot to the kid whose birthday it is." At yet another birthday party gathering, a grandmother there was reminiscing about her raising children days and commented, "I heard they don't even let you bring cupcakes to school anymore for your child's birthday."

Fruits and Seasons

Though fruit is obviously the better choice between itself (good sugar) and candy (not-good sugar), providing fruit for our children can prove difficult. Fresh, ripe fruit is expensive and takes more time and effort to have on hand, and that is why so many children don't get their daily fresh fruit. Families that have fruit trees in their yard are lucky. I search the markets for fruit. Although I don't like it, sometimes I'll spend five or six dollars for berries or even on one piece of fruit like a ripe cherimoya (an outrageously delicious fruit that I can only obtain when it's in season), because my daughter loves them. One day my husband, Michael, came home with expensive avocados. I said with incredulity, "You actually paid that much for each avocado?" They were really yummy. One day at my daughter's preschool afternoon snack, I noticed the large container of animal "crackers" (white flour and sugar cookies) from one of the Wal-Mart-like, bulk-buying stores. I figured the cookies costs about three dollars and that the container could last for maybe two or three weeks of snacks, while three dollars could not even purchase enough fresh fruit for one day's afternoon snack for the kids. Most daycares or preschools have to be reasonably priced so that parents can afford them. Consequently, childcare places cannot provide much in the way of quality, organic fruit and vegetables for the kids.

Knowing how to buy fruit is a special kind of knowledge that you learn over time. I used to not know much about different varieties of fruit, like when a particular fruit is in season, or ripe, and even today I'm still no fruit expert. Michael can pick up a watermelon, knock on it, and tell if it's any good inside. He's shown me how to do it a number of times, but I guess I'm tone deaf. I buy them and

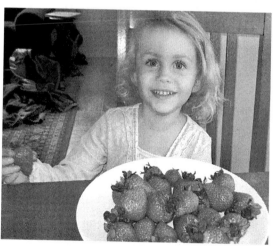 just hope for the best. Since Savanah's father is knowledgeable about fruit, Savanah has a keen sense about ripe fruit herself. One day her friend, Natasha, was over and went to pick an orangey-red strawberry from our garden. Savanah shrieked, "Don't eat it! It's not ripe." Many times I've cut into an avocado that wasn't ripe. They are hard, inedible, and since the avocado has been cut, it can no longer be put back on the shelf to ripen. I have no choice but to discard it. At three dollars or whatever the current rate happens to be per avocado, it's a bummer.

Raw foodists are serious about fruit, and some of them have contributed online video clips on Youtube.com about things like how to open a coconut or how to choose ripe avocados. Another nice website on fruit is TheFruitPages.com. I've learned a lot about fruit from going to the farmers markets and talking with the sellers. I focus on keeping the house stocked with fresh seasonal fruit, and keep dried and frozen berries on hand when fresh aren't available. I continue to be challenged by this, too, because I don't usually eat more than two pieces of fruit a day, and if Michael and Savanah don't eat it all, mandarins and peaches go to waste. And fruit is expensive.

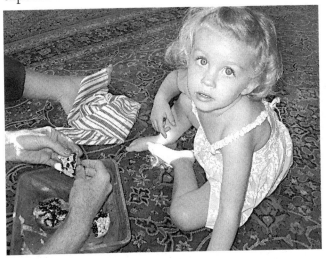

Daddy peeling a winter fruit, pomegranate, for Savanah.

Fruit out of season from distant lands doesn't make sense to me anymore. I used to regularly buy "fresh" berries in the store during the winter. I avoid this practice now because I am paying for the cost of the food's travel, fuel is wasted on transporting foods that are already available locally, and different methods of food transport encourage more pollution. We are already so sick because of such pollution. Also, health books constantly talk about the quality and actual nutritional value of 'traveling fruit.' By the time it gets to the table, its nutritional value is questionable. There's a huge difference between eating just-picked fruit and fruit that has been picked three days ago.

Still, feeding kids fruit instead of candy to satisfy their sweet demands, especially when holidays like Thanksgiving and Christmas start rolling around, is a better choice. Dried fruit works, but Savanah can't stand that stuff for the whole winter, and there's also the issue of sticky dried fruit and teeth. Feeding kids frozen fruit is questionable according to a few respected Eastern diet regimes that promote avoiding cold foods with kids as it slows the digestion process, but that's exactly what Savanah does for some sweet snacks—sits down to a bowl of straight frozen blueberries, cherries, and strawberries. I can buy frozen local berries during the winter. For the most part, berries are picked and frozen when they are ripe. Savanah can tell and spits out the fruit if it is sour tasting and not ripe. Frozen fruit may not be a best practice, but between watching Savanah eat a heap of candy and a heap of berries, I choose the latter. I do try to limit our fruit to what's in season and what's local.

Ice Cream and Juicers

There's no way to keep a child in the dark about ice cream. Pictures of ice cream paint repeatedly on the pages of children's books. My daughter literally started screaming for ice cream at about the age of two and a half. So far her idea of ice cream remains the kind we make in the Champion juicer with frozen fruit. There's a victory. Myself, if I'm going to go out and eat junk food, I rarely if ever go for ice cream. The ice cream made from frozen bananas and other frozen fruit like strawberries is extremely satisfying, tastes like ice cream, and many people say tastes even better than dairy ice cream. This ice cream comes from whole food, too, thus keeping the fiber and other nutrients in tact.

Juicers built to homogenize frozen fruit to make ice cream are awesome. Juicers prove easy to clean and assemble. It's just fruit going in so there's no scrubbing, just rinsing with hot water. It takes just about a minute to make ice cream! I use the Champion juicer and it is expensive, but I have also seen it on Craig's list. I consider the juicer a must-have kitchen item for kids. There are other high quality juicers available. Green Star is a serious, powerful juicer that stands as a notable brand, usually coming in first place for avid juicer users. It comes sturdy, already assembled, and stealthily hides its power cable in its body in the rear compartment. It uses stainless steel *twin gears* to crush the produce and expel the juice.

These gears are patented as they contain magnets and bioceramic materials in them, which are said to extract higher levels of minerals out of the produce and also give fresher juice with enzymes and vitamins that have a longer shelf life. Another product that works decently is called the Magic Bullet. Its seventeen piece kit includes with four party mugs, one tall cup, one short cup, the blender itself, one stainless steel flat blade, one stainless steel cross blade, two stay-fresh lids, and two shaker/steamer tops. In some reviews, it is criticized as being a blender more than a juicer, but it does the trick. Home juicing technology appeared in the 1950s. State of the art homogenizing came later and this may be the reason so many are not aware of this remarkable option. Children love sweet, frozen *licky things*. This kind of ice cream could be eaten for breakfast. No worries.

One day Savanah finally asked if we could go into the Baskin Robbins Ice Cream place that we pass on a regular basis. All the colors of the rainbow are there and happy smiling faces regularly flow from that place, so I knew it was just a matter of time. I was prepared. "No, Savanah. Baskin Robbins ice cream is made with high fructose corn syrup and that stuff is really bad for people and the planet." It worked. We're avoiding refined sugar, one day at a time.

For years I've dodged sugar and rainbow colored dyes used on the shaved ice served at the local farmers market. When Savanah was little and clueless, she would delight in the seasonally fresh strawberries and nectarines, which helped. As she's grown older, she has become increasingly more curious about foods. Then I began all kinds of strategies to avoid processed sugar. Not going to the market to avoid the shaved ice. At age five, she could have her choice of fresh cut flowers. Then I gave into her having the shaved ice without the dyes, followed by serious begging pressure and it got to be too big of deal for her. Now we do rainbow shaved ice, light on the syrup. Once something like shaved ice is introduced to a festival or market, it's hard to get it out. People come just for the junk food. Farmers markets across the country need to think seriously before they allow non-garden foods in. In the not-so-old days, garden food was all farmers markets had.

In the midst of supporting the effort to get a new library built in my neighborhood, one day I addressed the committee about our local fall library fundraiser, which was labeled as some sort of ice cream social. I asked if we could change the name to a Library Festival so the event wasn't so focused on the ice cream: "How about adding watermelon? It's in season at the same time." Nobody wanted to change the name as that was the signature name (though the event had happened once). I got much more involved and helped bring in more activities at the event, and then took the opportunity to try once again to get the group to change the name. I expressed to them, "For parents raising small children, we take our kids to support a new community library, and when the event's called an ice cream social, it makes the experience about ice cream." In the end, they modified the name, called it a festival, because it really is a festival now and the subtitle is an ice cream social and watermelon feed. Subtle changes add up.

I was impressed this last year at the library festival that they changed the literary cake walk (a game like musical chairs and the winner gets to take home a cake) so that the winners win a cupcake instead of dropping a whole cake on a family or kid. Despite all the great stuff happening at the event, the cupcake walk was Savanah's favorite part of the day.

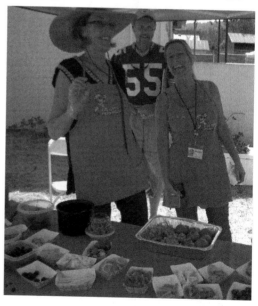

In addition, we added a booth for the school lunch program, where kids and adults alike could come make a potato head with a real potato and decorate with fresh fruits and veggies using tooth picks cut in half. At the same time, families could ask Kimberly about the lunch program. Pictured here from left is Deidre and Kimberly working the potato head booth.

Everywhere I see that most childcare providers and parents have fallen into the trap of rewarding and bribing kids with treats. Recently Savanah came home excited that if she learned her color words at preschool she would earn a purple or maybe orange ice cream cone. I have successfully avoided rewarding her with food or candy. If I do allow her to have candy, it's for no reason. When I first gave up white flour and sugar, I noticed how I searched for a reward after I did something amazing at work, a place where there is rarely appreciation or acknowledgement. In an effort to get relief without sugar, I once I got a manicure, but I to come to terms with myself without any consumption reward. The prize of food is deeply ingrained. I talked to Savanah's beautiful teacher about avoiding the use of food to reward Savanah. She said, "Yes, I haven't been using treats as reward. One of the parents gives a candy treat every time their child used the potty. Another older child started crying that it wasn't fair because she didn't get any candy so she just offered them something else to work on towards earning a candy reward." I recalled the old, simple gold star sticker tradition and what a good idea that is over candy.

The pink elephant in this discussion is parents' sugar habits, which is the number one factor for children's high sugar consumption. One mom told me she had her Ben & Jerry's ice cream hidden in a frozen vegetable bag for years. She thought the kids would never look in there. One day the kids got together and confronted her: "Mom, we know why you're chubby," and they thrust the half-eaten chocolate chip cookie dough ice cream at her. We have to deal with our own refined sugar habits as well as our kids. I know it's one of those much-easier-said-than-done realities. One option is to go to Twelve Step groups that deal with compulsive eating challenges and food addictions. Local meetings can be found on the Internet.

Savanah is almost six now and all the things I thought I'd never do, I've done. I've given her sugar-coated gum drop supplements. I've rewarded with candy and treats. The promise or denial of shaved ice grants me the behavior I most desire from Savanah. We make no tears muffins now. I've learned that it's better for me to make the muffins at home than to buy them at bakeries, as I sometimes found myself doing. I can make them with less sugar, fat, and preservatives, and with organic ingredients. The other day we made blueberry muffins, and for the half cup of sugar, I used a fourth of a cup of organic cane sugar and fourth of a teaspoon of Stevia, and Savanah enjoyed her muffin. Also, baking offers a tremendous amount of hands on science, math, and fun learning activities for kids. Last night I called out to Savanah, "Do you want to make corn bread with me?" She came running. As she pulled up her step stool she said happily, "Mommy, I love making stuff with you." As we mixed in the ingredients, Savanah got a lesson about fractions and the importance of exact measuring with baking in order to get the right tasting chemical reaction—the change of the combined liquid ingredients into a solid state. The kitchen is an important place in a child's life.

We all need to sacrifice sugar. With time, our muscle to resist temptation will grow. Less is more. We can offer less sugar at our children's birthdays. For example, we could try not to send kids home with a bag of candy from a birthday after they already had cake at the party. Community events and festivals can sell more wholesome foods with a smaller presence of ice cream and candy vendors. When we have other children over to our home, we can avoid not choosing baking cookies or cupcake decorating and eating as the main activity on an ordinary, non-birthday, nice weather day play date. We can plan ahead when we go places. We talk about how many treats our children can have at the amusement park, or parades, or anywhere else. We can bring snacks for our kids, because they are going to be hungry and what's immediately available might be deep-fried Twinkies. Each day that we can spare our children from refined sugar adds up to a longer, healthier life with healthy habits for them later on.

Fresh fruit is an economic trade off. For my family, in order to keep the fresh fruit regularly available around the house, it means we do and have less of other things. If the children of this great nation are going to get the daily fresh fruit that everyone agrees they need, and if we are going to subsidize the meat, dairy, and corn industries, which we do, then we need to also subsidize the fruit industry.

Teeth

Certain health-related subjects are too terrifying for me to read before bed. Teeth are one of them. One scary book called, *Root Canal Cover-Up: Exposed* argues that root canals are even worse than mercury fillings, and paints a picture as horrifying and poignant as Stephen King's novels. After becoming a parent, I started hearing more than a few dreadful stories about early childhood teeth trauma, and little did I imagine what my family's future would be.

For this book I started researching teeth and got in much further and deeper than I ever expected or desired. Now I notice young children with dental work, and I have a good idea what they've been through. Although not particularly sympathetic to the parental plight, one book that first woke me up some about teeth came from Dr. Herbert Shelton's *The Science and Fine Art of Food and Nutrition*. Dr. Shelton argued over a hundred years ago that teeth are bones and part of our skeletal system, and that the health of our teeth are mainly an inside job, meaning our diet contributes to the wellness of our teeth more than any amount of teeth brushing. Teeth are a big deal in scheme of health.

In our culture, we've become so good at making teeth look pretty that we've lost our way and understanding of how important healthy teeth are as part of the big picture of a strong body. Dental caries (cavities) are on the rise, and parents today have inherited a whole new level of teeth challenges. Tina, a local mother of three children tells her story about her first born: "My son had very serious decay at about eighteen months of age, which our MD doctor didn't identify at twelve months when I asked about white lines on his teeth. Grrrr. My son had to go under general anesthesia and get four root canals on his front top teeth as well as having them all capped and fillings in the other eight teeth he had at the time." (Note: the roots of milk teeth are not as deep and vast as adult teeth.)

Another mom summed it up well on our online parent group. After her four-year-old son had oral surgery, she wrote: "If you've ever had to deal with this you know there is always some guilt involved, like could we have prevented this if we brushed twice a day instead of one? Or given fluoride drops or not nursed so long... the list is endless."

Another parent said: "I felt so guilty, thinking I was a bad mom because of all of the crowns my son needed to get! It is genetic and weak teeth may just be a curse! One of the things that made his teeth worse was that he did nurse while sleeping, which has the same effects as milk bottles sorry to say to those who still nurse their toddlers in bed." Another mom argued back: "Actually, nursing for longer increases toddler's dental health. I think it is genetics, and some kids get more cavities than others."

Dr. Douglas Graham, author of *The 80 10 10 Diet*, addresses teeth in his book and has a short and excellent discussion on diet, dentistry and teeth available on youtube.com.[1] Here he tells a story about an intense program he went to with 70 other dentists and he asked four different dentists: What causes tooth decay? He got four different answers. The first one said it's because we eat too much fat. The second one said because we don't eat enough fat. Third one said because we eat too many carbohydrates. Fourth one said because we don't eat enough carbohydrates. And he basically suggests that first and foremost dentists are trained experts on working with teeth and health expertise falls more under the work of other doctors.

By the time children reach kindergarten, over forty percent of children already have one or more cavities.[2] Like many parents who get serious about researching teeth and their child's dental health, I sunk in deeper with the work of Dr. Weston Price, a dentist who did a landmark study around the 1920s to 1940s about the degeneration of teeth as caused by a modern diet. His work appears in his book, *Nutrition and Physical Degeneration*. He traveled remote

---

[1] http://www.youtube.com/watch?v=a0a8VWAtwMQ.

[2] http://pediatrics.about.com/od/nutrition/i/05_kids_raisins.htm According to the National Institute of Dental and Craniofacial Research

parts of the world to examine the teeth and diets of communities not yet touched by modernization. Price's question was: "Are there any groups of people who have healthy teeth and do not suffer from dental diseases?"

He found fourteen groups, tribes, or villages who had beautiful teeth, including room for wisdom teeth. He studied the Swiss, Eskimos, Native Indians, Aborigines, the Gaelic people, and other populations in around the world that had not yet had contact with modern foods. It was a critical time for his study as these segregated populations still existed but were quickly disappearing. Because of his astute timing in history, he was also able to document the quick degeneration of the teeth after people adopted "civilized" or a modern diet of processed foods. Photography was available at the time, enabling him to document what healthy teeth and faces look like. And no matter what the race, country or primitive diet, all the populations had remarkable things in common.

One commonality was that not one healthy group of people had a village dentist or tooth brushes either. Healthy, strong, and straight teeth were the norm. Dr. Price was also able to show that when people started eating modern, "white man's" foods, mainly processed foods, refined flours and sugars, and non-local whole foods, they quickly developed dental caries. Dr. Price demonstrated through photographs that physical degeneration began and was evident in only one generation after parents began eating a modern diet. The photographs show that people naturally had wider jaws, which allowed for the full set of teeth, and in just one generation that dental arch narrowed and teeth began to come in crowded. It was a horrendous time in dental history as the modern diet quickly transitioned in, and suddenly these people all over the world were plagued with dental caries and inflictions but had no dentists.

Today, normal and healthy teeth are rare. Unhealthy, weak, and crowded teeth are the standard. In addition to dentists, we have endodontists (root canal specialists) and orthodontists who concentrate on straightening teeth. Wisdom teeth are commonly pulled because our jaws have narrowed and there is no room for them to grow in properly. My dental hygienist reports that in just the last twenty years alone they are astounded by the number of children coming in with no wisdom teeth at all.

Price proved that malnutrition and diet is the *root* cause of dental caries. His landmark study gives parents the bigger picture of understanding that our children's dental problems are not just because they failed to use fluoride drops, brush two times a day or floss their teeth after meals. Our teeth are not separate from the rest of the body. Dr. Thomas S. Cowan writes in *The Fourfold Path to Healing*: "This is one of the evils that has accompanied modernization. We do not realize how much modern human beings are handicapped and injured since they learned how to modify Nature's foods.[3]" Cowan also writes that "Price's book is important for two reasons: One is that it shows, through the medium of photography, how healthy people look. They have broad faces, flawless straight teeth and muscular, well-formed physiques. Second, it describes the characteristics of their diets, which can be summed up in two words: **nutrient-dense** [emphasis mine]. None of the groups Dr. Price studied consumed a lowfat vegetarian diet, raw foods, and or practiced any system of food combining."[4] All these healthy tribes of people ate locally grown, whole foods wherever they lived in the world.

Still, what did those healthy-teeth people eat? *The Fourfold Path to Healing* and other present day related diet books have been written by Dr. Cowan, Sally Fallon, and other followers of Dr. Price, and these works promote a diet of raw dairy and meat from grass fed animals and soup made from the bones of these animals. Today, beef from free range cattle is not easily obtained, but the market seems to be growing rapidly and may become more prevalent in the near future.

A couple years ago I went to hear Victoria Boutenko speak, a well known mother and author in the raw food movement. Through raw foods, her family was able to restore their poor health, and her son avoided going on medication for diabetes. The whole family marveled at how quickly they felt well. In only four or so months of being on the 100% raw food diet; they ran races, hiked mountains, and wrote books about their new, remarkable life on a raw food diet. At one of her lectures promoting her latest book, Boutenko

---

[3] P. 494, Nutrition and Physical Degeneration, Weston A. Price

[4] P. 6, The fourfold Path to Healing, Thomas S. Cowan

stated that after about seven years, the whole family started having serious dental trouble. Holes began appearing right through their teeth.

She reported that her daughter didn't want to speak about raw foods anymore, saying she felt like a fraud. Boutenko said she knew the family couldn't go back to the Standard American Diet (SAD) because that was a dead end and so she firmly dove into research. Her studies took her to Jane Goodall's work and how the chimpanzees ate. From there, Boutenko began adding more greens to the family's diet. Her message in recent years has been a call to more greens. Because many of us no longer have the teeth strength and chewing power, she prescribes drinking green smoothies to get the greens that we need.

I met an old-timer, health educator, Arthur Andrews, at a local workshop and gathering on health, and he gave me his card. Nearly a year later when I came across his card again I gave him a call. He was eighty years old and had become bedridden since I had last seen him. He invited me to come visit him. During his last two years of bedridden but conversational life, I called on him regularly and he tried to download for me everything he knew and understood about health and living well. Arthur gave me all his dusty old books and cassette tapes of lectures he'd given and ones he'd attended. He was a generous person. Arthur had run a health sanctuary for a number of years where people did short and lengthy fasts. His health motto was:

"All raw food, organically grown, in modest portions and in proper combinations, lots of sunshine, fresh air, exercise, and positive thoughts."

I read and listened to Arthur's materials, hosting many parents who came long before me who studied natural foods in the modern age. Many tried eating a largely fruitarian diet, and the common thread I heard while listening to these tapes was that although they felt fabulous during the periods *that they were able to maintain* the diet, people commonly reported more sensitivity, discomfort in their teeth.

Having studied these parents and diets before I had a child, I was inspired to rear my child with good dental habits. Regularly, I'd brush Savanah's teeth or rinse her mouth after eating. I take care to clean off sticky dried fruit like figs, dates, Goji berries, raisins, or fruit leather. During the day when my daughter eats fruit and brushing isn't an option, I ask that she take a drink of water to rinse her teeth a little or I have her eat a celery stick.

Another guru writes that we've been conditioned to feed our babies soft foods. Many of us have anxiety from *the list* of foods that cause choking. Dr. Shelton wrote that teeth need exercising:

> "Soft diets, which require no work of the teeth and jaws in chewing, aid in producing dental decay. No tooth can have adequate nutrition unless it is used. Mush-eating does not give the teeth proper exercise. Raw foods are best. A tough, fibrous diet not only gives the teeth and jaws needed exercise, but also cleans the teeth. The conventional, unnatural and highly refined, cooked diet leaves the mouth and teeth dirty." [5]

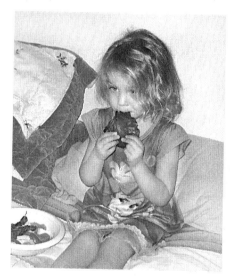

It's an interesting point Dr. Shelton makes that I have not read anywhere else. Who talks about exercising the teeth? I do recall how my dental hygienist once said she noticed that older people's health rapidly declines after they have all their teeth pulled for dentures. She said they no longer eat harder foods for the difficulty of chewing and fall into a diet of soft foods. Pictured here is Savanah snacking on red cabbage, jicama, carrots, and red pepper.

Fluoride

What is the deal with fluoride? Fluoride inflames major parental confusion on what is the right thing to do. Books like *The Fluoride Deception* and fluoride-free toothpastes continue to be produced while, at the same time, many doctors recommend fluoride prescriptions for our kids. Online, it is hard to find positive information about fluoride. *Scary information* is readily available.

I ran through *The Fluoride Deception* by Christopher Bryson. What I gathered was that the leading scientist, Phyllis Mullenix, who first led the extensive fluoride studies on rats showed that fluoride lowers their IQ and causes hyperactivity.[5] Maybe fluoride is the main culprit in the widespread attention deficit disorders among children? If so, are attention deficit disorders worth the hard enamel? I brought up my recent inquiry on fluoride with my sixty-something year old friend, Gemma. She grew up with die-hard holistic parents who did not allow her any junk food. The first thing out of her mouth was, "Rat poison." I understood where that came from.

Even the theory of how fluoride works appears to have changed recently. The Canadian Dental Association (CDA) no longer argues that "fluoride absorbed from the stomach via drinking water helps teeth."[6] Apparently, a new perspective is that the fluoride attacks via enzymes the cavity-causing bacteria in the mouth, but then, what about its effects on other vital chemical catalysts in the mouth and in the body?

While reading online about fluoride, a name kept coming up: Dr. Hardy Limeback. He is a leading Canadian fluoride authority and expert who is often cited by health officials in their defense of fluoridated water. He is also a long-standing consultant to the Canadian Dental Association and a professor of dentistry at the University of Toronto. Recently, he has conceded that "fluoride may be destroying our bones, our teeth, and our overall health."[7] Although he still believes fluoride in toothpaste is effective against tooth decay, he says it doesn't need to be added to our water and we may be taking unnecessary risks by doing so. Dr. Hardy Limeback says: "Almost all the beverages we drink (beer, pop, juice) are made with fluoridated water. Fish and other foods also contain fluoride. Many of the vegetables we eat are fertilized with compounds containing fluoride; they are irrigated with, and washed and cooked in, fluoridated water. So we are getting far more fluoride than it appears.

---

5 P.17, The Fluoride Deception, Christopher Bryson

6 P.xix-xx, The Fluoride Deception, Christopher Bryson

7 http://www.actionpa.org/fluoride/torontostar.html

A Dr. Lee has also established a direct link between fluoride use, osteoporosis and increased incidence of hip fractures in his report, *A Brief Account of the Fluoridation and Hip Fracture Problem*.[8]

Limeback also writes: "Contrary to popular belief, there is no proof that fluoride fights cavities. In the U.S., the government recently ordered toothpaste manufacturers to stop claiming it does until they could prove it." There's a new warning label now on the back of fluoridated toothpaste that reads: "WARNINGS: Keep out of reach of children under 6 years of age. If you accidentally swallow more than used for brushing, seek professional help or contact a poison control center immediately." Though we don't want our kids going around spitting, we have got to teach them to be great spitters with toothpaste. At four and a half years old, Savanah can barely spit. At what age should kids use fluoride toothpaste while early childhood decay is so prevalent?

Amalgams

There are numerous books that address mercury toxicity and amalgams. An amalgam is a mixture of mercury, silver, copper, tin, and zinc, and mercury comprises the largest portion at around fifty percent.[9] Given an option, what informed parent would allow a dentist to fill their child's teeth with an amalgam filling? I've heard mercury is the most deadly substance on the planet. It seems that because it is cheap, durable, and long established, the American Dental Association (ADA) has still not banned the use of amalgams.

Many dentists have been in battle amongst themselves over the use of mercury since 1840. Dentist, author and activist, Dr. Hal A. Huggins compares the ADA and its unwillingness to inform patients of its use of toxic substances like mercury to the automobile industry when it fought against the mandatory installation of seat belts. "The implication was that you could get hurt in a car. The admission of this obvious fact led to the saving of thousands of lives every year due to the presence of seat belts."[10]

---

[8] http://www.cuprident.com/fluoride.php

[9] P. 23, *It's All In Your Head*, Dr. Hal A. Huggins

[10] P. 19, It's All In Your Head, Dr. Hal A. Huggins

Today, many dentists continue to use amalgams, and loads of parents do not understand that their child's teeth are being filled with this highly controversial material unless they ask their dentist. However, one dentist office we patronize, which hosts three different dentists, has not used amalgams for thirty years. But, before anyone goes rushing out to get all their amalgams out, my husband suffered major jaw pain and endured years of dental problems following a decision to have all his amalgam fillings removed. He suggests not having any dental work unless there's trouble.

Savanah's First Teeth Cleaning

When Savanah turned three, I had my dentist take a quick look at her teeth. At four-and-a-half, she went for her first official teeth cleaning and checkup. It took significant preparation to get Savanah to cooperate with the dentist. She sat and watched me get my teeth cleaned and the reality exposure didn't help any. Twice, she watched a muppet-like video with real children enacting a fun, authentic trip to the dentist, which she enjoyed watching. Full force bribery was activated in order to get her to collaborate peacefully. She would get to go swimming afterwards. She could finally earn a princess book she had been longing for, and, if she didn't oblige, she would have her two new beloved swimming suits taken away for a day. She cooperated beautifully. The hygienist said "open wide like an alligator," and she did. Savanah bought into the mouth vacuum with the name, "Mr. Thirsty." And in the car ride home she said, "Mommy, I loved going to the dentist! I could go everyday!"

The hygienist gave big thumbs up for the liberal space between each tooth on the top of her mouth. She said when the teeth are spaced too closely; it is harder for the new teeth to come in nicely. Although her bottom teeth are straight and not crowded, the nice spacing that's happened on the top isn't occurring on the bottom.

While polishing her teeth, the hygienist noted a stain or possibly some decay, but said the dentist would have to check and let us know. Fear grabbed me by the shoulders. My stomach tightened. Inwardly I begged, "No, please!" A good looking, youthful and jet-black haired Persian dentist came in. (I've met three Persian dentists in the past year. Do Persian mothers encourage their children to become dentists? If so, smart. Talk about job security!) The dentists quickly finessed Savanah to open like an alligator while he counted her twenty teeth. The decision was announced: Decay. It was the end of my world.

The dentist said he could repair the decay quickly without having to put her under and without any Novocain. Having heard the horror stories, I was grateful it wasn't more serious.

"What if we didn't do anything?" I asked, searching for hope.

The hygienist replied, "Then it would get bigger and there would be tooth aches."

I searched my options. "What if the tooth was pulled?" I asked.

"The tooth next to it would lean in the open space and then the new tooth couldn't come in properly," she said.

Regressing to my drugs-to-fix-problems mentality, I asked about the fluoride prescriptions and the controversy around fluoride.

The hygienist dismissed it. "There's controversy over everything. I gave my daughter fluoride and she's never had a cavity. It's really too late now to take fluoride to help with the development of the enamel. I think she's old enough where she is able to spit toothpaste out. You don't want them swallowing the fluoride. The toothpaste won't help systemically, but may help some on the surface."

I got the message that our time was up. I left the office wondering. How come it's safe to take fluoride prescriptions but toxic to swallow fluoride tooth paste? My mind went haywire and I told myself, "Even though I might be poisoning her, I should have given her the fluoride drops."

Feeling somber, I chauffeured the clueless, tooth-decay Savanah to the swimming pool. I took my inventory. I thought, who cares if I would have looked obsessive, I should have carried her beloved Hello Kitty toothbrush in my back pocket and shoved it in her mouth after every snack. Maybe the decay started in the womb when her teeth buds were forming and I made those four trips to Denny's for French toast and maple syrup. She sucked on orange slices the first two years of her life. Forget all the great vitamin C, the citrus acid weakened her enamel. I thought harder. The decay is on her right side. She nursed herself to sleep every night on my left; that means if the milk pooled in her mouth it would have stagnated on the right-side of her mouth, the side that's decaying.

Price proved that in leaving nature and natural foods behind, we have led ourselves into a multi-generation of dental degeneration. Nursing is one of the few remaining natural things that some of us do. I've never had any trouble with putting Savanah to bed because I have nursed her at night. No ugly go-to-bed battles. Maybe the decay is because of the night time nursing? I find that a hard one to swallow. Nursing is more than just sustenance. I learned to believe along the way that the act of nursing by the child develops the jaw and face. "Sucking at the breast uses more muscles than sucking on a bottle nipple and leads to better development of the face, the mouth, and the tongue, which give teeth a better chance to grow in straight. Dr. Sears said, "In a study of ten thousand children. Those who were breastfed for a year or more were forty percent less likely to require orthodontic treatment.[11] But some people are not saying to give up nursing, just night time nursing. But separating the two is easier said than done for me. When I later asked a well seasoned lactation consultant and nurse about dental caries and nursing she responded, "I don't buy it. Some kids just have weak teeth and others don't."

The fact of the matter is, Savanah has had processed white flour and sugary foods, sometimes at the hand of Michael, me, or the outside world; not every day or every week, and generally began after she turned three-and-a-half when she started preschool, and was cognizant of Halloween, the winter holidays and birthdays. Dr. Price proved that the refined sugar and flour are (and always have been) the first culprits. Her diet has been considerably better than average for eating whole foods and less candy than most kids. At the same time, Savanah's eaten a lot of dried fruit, especially over the winter, and it often didn't follow by immediate brushing. Sticky raisins, figs or other sweets don't come off easily and left to sit on the back teeth—it's just not good. Dentists don't promote raisins and the like for kids.

---

[11] P.240, The Family Nutrition Book, Dr. Sears

I've brushed Savanah's teeth with just water, because she can't spit, religiously every night before bed. Usually in the morning or sometime in the day she gets another brushing, but I could have brushed her teeth more. I floss her teeth sometimes so she would get used to it. Michael and I both love our floss. I bust through a bag of floss sticks a month! I figured Savanah is getting great flossing role models. Certainly, I could have done more or brushed her teeth better when I did. In reflection, I would say to another mom who took my same actions: "You've been more than responsible!"

Savanah has inherited her teeth from Michael and me. We both have narrow jaws and mouths full of fillings. I didn't have any early childhood decay and my diet was worse than hers. I drank fluoridated water and used fluoride tooth paste. When I was in eleventh grade, wham my dentist told me I had eleven cavities. I've read that the teenage years are another sensitive period where caries occur more easily, so it's important to remind teenagers about brushing and flossing. Despite the well known junk food teenage diet today, so many more young people now are health-conscious and smart these days about taking care of their bodies.

Although I see Savanah as having almost extraordinary health, I am wondering about adequate nutrition because now I view the teeth as part of the whole and not something separate from the body. I'm concerned.

At home, I went over the dental details with Michael, who is as up on dentistry if not more so than I. As a young adult, he had all his mercury fillings removed. Although many people have their mercury fillings removed without any trouble, what followed for Michael were years of excruciating jaw pain and trips to various dentists to get his teeth and jaw lined up correctly. I told him, "I called four different dentists that have distracting equipment for kids like playing Dora videos on the ceiling or putting on special video-playing goggles on while dental work is done, but all the local, high-tech children dentists I could find are not taking new patients. I'm glad that the work can be done without drugs but I'm concerned about the work being too much for her." Thoughtfully, Michael responded, "Of course I'm not happy about the decay, but the experience may be helpful to Savanah's maturation process. I want her to be present with the dental work and not be distracted. Just take her to our regular dentist to have the work done." I think to myself, "and who's going to be the one at the dentist office going through this experience and holding her hand? Me." I acquiesce to his wishes because I am reminded of the words of Michio Kushi, the famous Macrobiotic teacher and author:

> "Often, especially in modern society, parents' love and care for their children takes a sentimental orientation. Children are protected from all hardships including cold weather, material poverty, social misery, and various other difficulties. Such artificial separation from life's adversities tends to spoil children's development of self-discipline, endurance, vitality and understanding."[12]

The evening following her trip to the dentist and to Savanah's glee, Michael and I took turns playing dentist with Savanah. I laid myself down in a lawn chair and opened my mouth like an alligator. "Mr. Thirsty" was a straw in a glass of water. When I finished, I was able to pick a prize.

When I thought about the families and little ones just in my neighborhood, I figured we were at fifty percent for dental caries in preschool age kids. I decided to look it up. In my own estimate, early childhood tooth decay is at epidemic proportions. In a May 10, 2007 ADA report online entitled, "Caries rate climbs for toddlers," doctors report:

> "'Sadly, tooth decay in our youngest population—kids 2-5—has increased about 4 percent over the last 10 years. All of America should be concerned with this statistic,' says Dr. Roth.

> "'The news of increasing decay in baby teeth is distressing,' said Dr. Vincent Filanova, chair, ADA Council on Access, Prevention and Inter-professional Relations. The dental community will be stepping up with strong educational activities to encourage young families to recognize the importance of early tooth brushing habits, flossing and

---

12 P. 139, The Book of Macrobiotics, Michio Kushi

eating healthy food choices along with a child's first dental visit before their first birthday."[13]

I didn't want to think about teeth anymore. There was too much anguish around the subject. I recall the saying: "Ignore your teeth and they'll go away." I'm no different from all the other loving parents out there. I want my kid to have strong and healthy teeth.

A week later, we took Savanah to our new dentist. I've noticed this dentist is x-ray happy. He takes before and after shots. It's no surprise to me that he wants to get an x-ray of Savanah's right and left sides to see in between her teeth. He shoved an adult size cardboard backdrop in her little four and a half year old mouth and while she choked and her eyes teared up, he got a picture of her right side. He tried to put it in again on the other side, and she screamed so loud that the lady in the dental chair on the other side of the partition let out a startled scream in response. I cheered Savanah on, "You can do this!" Michael, taking off work to help, gave me a silencing hand and interjected calmly, "Daddy promised when you're done he would take you to the toy store and get you a Hello Kitty." All Savanah had to do was hold that thing in her mouth and feel like she was choking to death for ten seconds. At four and half, she doesn't have the development to understand this. She is in survival mode. We all agreed it was time to call it a rap before she was totally traumatized. Daddy headed for the toy store anyway.

The dentist said Savanah was going to lose the tooth next to her front teeth that clearly had a cavity, so we just need to watch it. That same tooth is the one I had my dentist take a look at when she was three because it had a small indentation in it. I think it just came in weak. Interestingly, the dentist suggested putting sealants on her back baby teeth because they don't come out until she's about ten. I didn't realize they could do that. I thought they did that when the permanent molars come in at five or six. In this way, he said, they could clean off the plaque that's started on the back right side and put sealants on them. This sounded better than having a filling.

---

[13] http://www.ada.org/prof/resources/pubs/adanews/adanewsarticle.asp?articleid=2493

Two weeks passed before we returned to the dentist. This time a young female dentist, with a dazzling smile and designer shoes, came out for Savanah. The dentist informed me that she was going to have me sit in the waiting room. Fine with me. If you can get the job done without me, great. I peeked around the corner and saw that they put "Harold and the Purple Crayon" DVD I brought on the television, one of Savanah's favorites. I wanted her to have something familiar and comforting. For twenty minutes I was in the waiting room, sneaking looks around the corner at her, and I was so proud. She was cooperating. She was being brave. I didn't hear crying. She had serious motivation, a new singing Barbie. I looked around the waiting room at the one-of-a-kind works of art: original paintings, sculptures, Turkish rugs. I was reminded of the children's book series, "Fancy Nancy." The place was posh. There was a small refrigerator for patients with bottled sparkling water, juice and Frappacinos. Business was good. I looked at the family photos and noticed they were Persian, too.

The beautiful, dark haired, young dentist came out. "I'm afraid we haven't been able to do anything. I got the surfaces cleaned off and ready but she keeps putting her tongue in the way and she's reached her threshold. I feel that she'll be traumatized if we go any further," she said. I told the dentist, "I've got a singing Barbie in the car that I'll go get and come in and hold her hand. Let's give it one more try to see if you can finish the job on the right side." We tried, and to my dismay, Savanah couldn't stop her tears or from moving her tongue in the way of the doctor.

The doctor referred us to a pediatric dentist, and suggested that she be put under to have the sealants put on. Savanah accepted that she wouldn't get the singing Barbie. Michael didn't take the news well of having her put under. Michael called the 'posh' dentist, talked with them about Savanah's "visit" and asked me to make an appointment with the pediatric dentist.

And so, we joined the flawed ranks of the many parents facing early-child tooth decay. The challenges have been formidable. These caries come largely from generations of the modern diet and current practices. Dr. Meinig, author of the *Root Canal Cover-Up: Exposed*, said in an online interview that sums up some of my conclusions from researching teeth:

"During the last sixty or more years we have added in increasing amounts, highly refined and fabricated cereals and boxed mixes of all kinds, soft drinks, refined vegetable oils and a whole host of other foodless 'foods'. It is also during those same years that we as a nation have installed more and more root canal fillings—and degenerative diseases have become rampant. I believe—and Dr. Price certainly proved to my satisfaction—that these simultaneous factors are *not* coincidences."

And in regard to oral hygiene Dr. Meinig says, "Of course, hygiene practices are preventive, and help minimize the destructive effect of our 'civilized,' refined diet. But the real issue is still diet. The natives Dr. Price tracked down and studied weren't free of cavities, inflamed gums, and degenerative diseases because they had better tooth brushes. It's so easy to lose sight of the significance of what Dr. Price discovered. We tend to sweep it under the rug—we'd actually prefer to hear that if we would just brush better, longer, or more often, we too could be free of dental problems."

Two weeks later, we arrived at the third dentist, a pediatric office. The balloons, promises for prizes, cute sayings all worked their magic on Savanah. She talked with them easily, but then it came time to lie back in the chair and open her mouth. She tightened up like twisted rope. She didn't want to cooperate. The dentist said, "I'm only going to count your teeth." He counted on her fingers. She relaxed for a moment, but as soon as he touched his poking hand tool down on a tooth she froze. I chimed in about the singing Barbie waiting for her if she cooperated. She opened wide but was only able to maintain her courage for a moment before she started to shake and her eyes filled. The last place I wanted to be was here. In a harsher, straight-forward tone I uttered, "You've got to do this or you're not getting the singing Barbie. He's not going to do anything but look at your teeth." The dentist could barely get through a physical tooth exam, let alone an X-ray.

We talked for five minutes afterwards about our options. One, he said that he didn't use the syrup medication to relax kids because a dentist has to monitor the child at the same time he's working on their teeth, and he feels it's too much to pay attention to blood pressure and vitals when you get focused on working on the teeth. He said they use an anesthesiologist. Because she is healthy, the risks for her are extremely low. He used the old *more likely to get in a car accident* comparison than die from being put under. He said he couldn't tell what was really going on with those brown stains on top of her back right teeth. He needed an X-ray. All three dentists have said that they needed X-rays. He said that it's just the way it is: some children and even some adults gag on the mouth piece for taking X-rays. We should come back in three or four months when she has a little more maturity on her and to see if we could get an X-ray.

For three months after the visit, we went through the holiday season, which brought a few more sweets, and I found that I felt discouraged. All my best efforts and vigilance had not saved my child from tooth decay. I caved into Savanah's request for a little something sweet here and there. "You have cavities," I told her. "We must not have treats too often." She said, "I don't want cavities." I said, "Nobody does, honey."

We went over to our friend's house. I noticed Savanah and her little friend, Alana, are quiet downstairs. I went down to check on them. They were in the bathroom and Alana, who is bribed with candy (out of home-office working mom's desperation) and has a real sweet tooth, was sucking down the grape or whatever sweet flavored toothpaste, while Savanah curiously eyed her like she was waiting for her turn. I interrupted them and was glad to know that their mother used some Chinese herbal product and that they weren't ingesting large quantities of fluoride. I didn't have to call the poison control hotline.

Three months later, the dreaded dentist appointment was upon us. I wished Michael didn't have to work and I could turn this job over to him. I promised Savanah a trip to the nearby toy store after the visit if she would cooperate. I hid a surprise stuffy (she's wild for any soft, cute stuffed doll or animal) in my purse to pull out for inspiration.

She was in the chair. She dreamt of all the promised rewards. I pulled out the surprise stuffy to rally her on. She couldn't do it. Crestfallen and angry, I left the room and hoped the dentist could work a miracle with her without me. Ten minutes later, they came and got me. They couldn't get an X-ray. The dentist told me instead of three or four possible cavities, she now had possibly five or six.

Five or six! Now she must be put under to have X-rays, filling and sealants. I told myself that she could at least sit in the chair at this age and be pleasant with the staff, she just couldn't endure stuffed things in her mouth. I asked the dentist about fluoride. He named a common mouthwash, which has a very low fluoride level.

On the way home, I bought a bottle of the mint-flavored mouthwash and soaked Savanah's "Dora the Explorer" toothbrush in it, and brushed her teeth. She loved the taste. For the moment, she likes getting her teeth brushed. Yum. Although I was not comfortable with the stuff, I was less comfortable with giving her an oral prescription to ingest. What did I know? Our darling friends have been giving their daughter of the same age a fluoride prescription, and she has no cavities and does not have to be put under of which I am very glad for them.

One morning as Savanah awoke, I held her close and noticed how strong her breath smelled. I smiled to myself thinking that even my child's bad breath did not bother me. I love her completely. Shortly afterwards, Michael said to me, "Do you notice how bad her breath is in the morning?" I nodded. He went on, "I'm concerned. A child's breath shouldn't be so strong. She's sick, Sue." I responded, "It may be the stench of rotting teeth. I will look up online halitosis and children. I am concerned, too. If her teeth have cavities, and teeth are not separate from her body, how well is she?" Michael and I reviewed her diet and concluded that we could not see much that we could do differently.

The next day I looked up halitosis online (the condition of having stale or foul-smelling breath) and found that childhood halitosis is indeed connected with dental caries. I also went to the store and bought some candy-like calcium supplements for kids. Everywhere we read about calcium and teeth but all we're given is that dairy products provide the needed calcium, but dairy isn't doable for what seems is a fast growing many, and then in that case, we should take a supplement? I looked at the rice and almond milk Savanah drinks. They both have about thirty-five percent RDA of calcium and significant amounts of sugar. If she's got "weak" teeth, then maybe we need to be more rigorous about calcium, but how effective are they?

Michael and I read the literature on the procedure for putting Savanah under. Neither of us could fully understand the combination of gas used and medicine injected. And although we carry some of the best dental insurance available today, we have to come down with a $1,000.00 deposit and insurance will only cover the cost of amalgams.

A week before the appointment, Michael and I had a cleansing fight. One point of contention brought up was that Daddy went to meet with the dentist for an hour last Saturday so that he could be informed about Savanah going under. "Do you realize all the decisions that need to be made while she's under? Why didn't you do more of the leg work and research?" he demanded. "I'm already working sixty hours a week," I said, "And I've been resenting all these office visits." I realized then that any sick child builds up a tension in the parents. Everywhere parents must fight over their ailing children. Who's responsible? Who's to blame? The airing of feelings gave me the strength to step up to the plate once more and face this dental nightmare along with Michael. I felt it wouldn't be fair to "check out" and leave Daddy to do this tough job alone.

We stayed up late the night before so Savanah would sleep later because she could not eat before her ten o'clock appointment. We waited an hour in the waiting room while "Wall-E" played on the TV screen. Michael played trains with her on their train table. The tall, fit anesthesiologist came into the waiting room to get us. If I had worn a skirt, Savanah would have been under it. She wasn't crying, but she was afraid.

We went into a small room with one dental chair. The anesthesiologist had all his portable equipment dressed up like Christmas. The tubes looked like candy canes, there was a Rudolph the Red-Nosed Reindeer, and his nose lit up. I wanted to tease him later about how un-politically correct this was but I checked myself as I shouldn't have been joking at a time like this. Michael had been instructed to retain Savanah in his arms in her "crisscross apple sauce" position as soon as they were underway. The doctor gave Daddy a mask, himself and Savanah one to breathe. "Smells like bubblegum!" he said. Suspiciously she lightly held it to her face. Swiftly and aggressively the doctor slammed the mask to her face and locked it into position with a jarring hand grip under her jaw.

Her eyes riveted toward me. She flailed. She fought like one trying to save her life from people who were trying to kill her. The doctor assured us, "she's already not remembering this."

The sight was terrible to watch. My eyes watered up. After about a minute, the doctor took her from Michael. She was snoring for the first time in her life and he said this is normal. Again, he quickly and aggressively executed medical procedures. Shoved a tube up her nose and in her veins. All the time he was talking to us and telling us what he was doing. Michael got up and moved to end of the chair to get out of the way. His face was white. I felt his energy. He was close to passing out. His body swayed from having to hold his little girl down and feel her fight for her life. I quickly got a rolling stool from the dental office and put my hand on him, trying to ground him. He sat on the stool, dropped his head between his knees, and forced himself to breathe. It seemed that the worst part was over.

An eight-month pregnant Vietnamese dentist waddled into the room and carried out the X-rays. All in all, Savanah had nine cavities. Nine! All eight back teeth, top and bottom had decay in between. Apparently, if one side gets it, the tooth next to it easily becomes "infected." The dentist said that Savanah has unusually deep and well-defined groves in her milk (baby) teeth like that of adult teeth, and this factor makes it extremely difficult to get in there. Then I had one fleeting moment of relief. She said something to the effect that this is probably the leading reason for the dire situation, and there was nothing we could have done to make things different. (Later my hygienist said that's where the fluoride helps to make the enamel thicker and grooves less defined.)

The two doctors offered up, "At least Savanah will not lose any teeth. Many children have to have extractions done." Then the dentist talked about the six-year-molars that will be coming only a year away. I wondered if I could maintain an obsessive compulsive brushing and flossing routine. The dentist continued to ask me questions and talk with me after that and I found that I wanted to leave the room because, although she could work like a carpenter and talk and work at the same time and I could talk for hours about children and dentistry work now, I wanted her to focus on what she was doing.

When it was all over, the dentist gave me a low dose fluoride prescription. Of course, I was ready to give her any magic pill promise. Michael said, "Find me some support, some studies to back it up and I'll be okay with it." It's hard to get access to Dental journals and the like on the Internet without paying membership fees, so I went looking at my dentist office. My hygienist said, "The fluoride now will make her wisdom teeth stronger. All the other teeth are already formed." I was surprised then when a young dentist in the office came in next and responded, "I would never give my child fluoride to ingest. It's poison."

The next day I found myself feeling angry. One, my daughter and I went out into the world and she was given candy. Two, I found I could easily add fuel to my anger by thinking about the anesthesiologist, who charged by the minute the highest rate I ever heard for anything. I understood training and malpractice insurance, but geez. This fit, middle-aged young man wasn't crawling under a house to get the job done. Rather, he was making brief calls on his cell phone and texting because my little one was safely snoring away. That was just *his* fee. There were all the ladies in the office, the expensive dentist doing the actual work, and not to mention all the insurance people who have to be involved.

In the end, Savanah woke up shocked, dismayed and angry. She wanted that silver crown in the back of her mouth out. Even two months later, she expressed her sadness about having it.

Afterwards and one day while swimming in our community pool, I noticed a smiley, young boy, around the age of four, with all four front teeth pulled and some silver caps in the back. I struck up a conversation with the mother. "I see your son had to have some dental work like my daughter." (It doesn't take much to get a parent to start talking about their kid.) She began with the dentist who did the work and how he used the sedating drink. She said she breastfed and used the prescription fluoride drops. She has an older child, so she knew to clean and brush from tooth number one. She had cavities as a child. The father did not. The tops of her son's teeth started showing gray decay at 18 – 24 months. She said, "His decayed teeth had to be pulled, otherwise they would have damaged his permanent teeth. It cost us thousands of dollars out of pocket and that was with insurance." I asked her about her diet while she was pregnant. The healthy, not overweight-looking mom said, "I worked at a health food store while I was pregnant with him. I don't eat a lot of meat, but I feel like I ate well, and I took all the prenatal vitamins and the omegas." Neither of us could think of anything she could have done differently.

In addition to our plain just not knowing what more to feed our children in their ever hungry, growing state, many of us have this general belief: "I ate sugary cereals for breakfast and cookies every night and I turned out okay." I've come to the conclusion that this early childhood teeth problem is an argument against this belief. Even with astute care to nutrition and caring for early teeth, many caries can't be prevented because of lifelong diets in parents and past generations.

Savanah has a new chance with her permanent teeth. While my daughter and I travel about in our daily lives, now I carry xylitol gum for a quick chew in the car after eating, for example, a burrito or some fruit if we won't be stopping to brush her teeth. I'm not keen on gum as it's also another stimulant and habit that I'm introducing, but the Xylitol neutralizes bad bacteria in the mouth. Savanah's going to need time and her own tooth brush and supplies to care for her teeth at school. She's not going to want to miss recess time like the other kids. How can she take care of her teeth during the full school day? Given the new rapid rise in early childhood tooth decay, we must now respond and adjust our school schedules to incorporate and allot time for the option of children to care for their teeth. I am happy that I am currently around after kindergarten for Savanah just so I am able to brush her teeth after lunch and during the day. She still isn't very good at brushing her own teeth, and no one or program out in the world is able to give her this attention that she and many others most definitely need.

Not unlike how western medicine went overboard with penicillin after its discovery, my understanding is that we did the same with fluoride and the consequences are far reaching and complex. Further, I understand that fluoride is toxic, but it's the only band aid we know today that apparently helps build thicker enamel, which might be a necessary evil because of the modern diet of most children.

Every night we have a routine that neither Savanah nor I enjoy but accept. She sits on top of the toilet with the cover down, and I squat below trying to see inside her tiny mouth. "Open up, Savanah," I say feeling already impatient. She exaggerates and opens her mouth as wide as she possible can, to the point where it hurts her to have it open that wide. I am able to floss a few teeth. Then we have to pause. All of sudden a child who has no trouble sitting still at school, cannot sit still for three seconds. Her head is twisting and her body bobbing. "*Please*, Savanah," I beg her. She opens her mouth. I get the floss between three sets of tight molars and there's one spot in the far back of her mouth where I have trouble feeling or seeing if I got the floss in it or not. As I push up too hard in that space Savanah growls, "You got it!" "Okay," I huff back. When the evening's flossing and brushing is over, we are both relieved and happy again.

Growing and Gathering Food

Many of us learned about the food pyramid in school, but how many of us ever learned the basics? As an adult I knew more about international cuisines from various countries, e.g., Thai, Indian, and Korean, yet what was my knowledge of local foods and ingredients like kohlrabi, when mandarins are in season, or how long the planting season for peas is? Teaching children in their earliest years about whole foods, seasonal varieties, and gardening are fundamental life skills, and one of the best ways to nurture a nuanced understanding of locally accessible produce is to have children shop for food and grow it themselves.

Shopping For Food

One of four children, I was usually the one to accompany my mother grocery shopping every Saturday. I suggested meal ideas while we shopped, and I was happy to help her with the loading and unloading of groceries. My mother was passionate about sewing, not food and cooking, but I'd like to think that she liked shopping with me as much as I did with her. We got our flat bed grocery cart and idly scanned the aisles of the food warehouse. The boxed and canned foods, the cashiers, the smells, the displays were utilitarian and unexceptional. The whole atmosphere reflected well how my mother felt about the whole business of piling up on provisions for her family to make it through another week.

Given some early training, how come shopping for food seems so complex to me now? For one, I eat significantly different than I did growing up, e.g.: I ate meat and potatoes and hardly any beans. Two, there weren't health food stores or farmers markets in our area. We would only stop at road side produce stands for strawberries or corn in the summer. Three, there weren't so many choices and places to shop for food. Four, there was little thought or added complexity about buying organic, non GMO,[1] local and little awareness about packaging or additives. And there are even more reasons why shopping for food might take more thought, concentration, and effort today.

I find that in order to eat the most economical, organic fresh fruits and vegetables everyday, I have to shop more than twice a week.

Within twenty minutes from my home, there are different kinds of places to shop for necessities, and I hit all of them throughout the year. Sometimes I hit a flea market looking for fruit or other food deals, and schlep cases of mangos or oranges home. Then once in a while I tag along with a friend who has a Costco (super store) membership, and buy a five pound bag of organic, short grain brown rice or other mass quantity foodstuffs. Costco has everything

[1] A **genetically modified organism (GMO)** is an organism whose genetic material has been altered using genetic engineering techniques (Wikipedia).

from clothes, furniture, toys, meat, and nearly every kind of food, frozen, boxed, and fresh. I don't like to go much because I find that it's a Herculean task for me not to impulse buy there.

I stop at the large, local, common chain stores like Safeway and use my buyers' club card to save money, and maybe contribute to my local school during their fundraising periods. How is it possible to save so much using their member tracking card? They must mark up the prices on the club buyers stuff to make me *feel* like I'm getting such a deal. Maybe I should get some handheld electronic device to help me remember how much a bag of pasta costs at store x in order to be able to look it up when I'm at store y, because I can't keep all these prices in my head.

I go to a farmers market every week. One reason is to stay in tune with the foods that are in season—to get at that "eat a wide variety of fresh fruits and vegetables" goal that I never quite know if we've reached. I also go because every food purchase is a vote. Jane Goodall writes in her book, *Harvest for Hope*, "Buying your food from a local farmer who is a good steward of the earth is one of the most effective contributions you can make to the health of the planet." The produce has recently been picked. Farmers market food hasn't traveled from across the country or come from another continent. Buying produce from a farmers market supports local jobs and businesses that do not use toxic chemicals that get into our water and soil. I also find most of the people working at the markets to be kind, hard working, and pleasant souls.

Imported Versus Local

I used to go regularly to the large local chain store, Safeway, for organic, fresh blueberries on sale during the winter until I read the label. They're coming all the way from South America. Because I want to reduce pollution caused by excessive food travel, I try to avoid participating in those purchases. I decided that it's better to stay with locally grown frozen ones during the winter. Bananas are hard to give up, but I'm learning my list while living in California is pretty small for foreign foodstuff needs, like the frozen pizza and packaged pasta from Italy sold at Trader Joe's, which is preposterous particularly with pizza, which is made locally everywhere in the U.S.

Trader Joe's is the place where a lot of savvy, health conscious shoppers go for saving money while adding more natural foods to their diet. Sometimes the difference between an organic product at Trader Joe's and the local health food store can be really significant. My friend, Paula, who has mastered the art of bargain shopping once said, "For the same amount of money, I can walk out of Trader Joe's with twice the amount of groceries than I can at New Leaf (the health food store)." I've never been comfortable about how everything at Trader Joe's is packaged. For convenience, I guess, they don't use any scales so nearly all the products have to be in some sort of package. I also find myself buying a lot of organic junk food there, like "Baked Snap Peas" for Savanah. There's not much difference between these and a bag of potato chips, but "Baked Snap Peas" sounds healthier. I go there because I can no longer afford to solely buy my goods and products from my local health food store, and I don't know many families that can.

Finding a good balance between low-priced, good quality, and earth-friendly products can be tricky—it's like juggling. I spend a good deal of time shopping at multiple venues. Whole, organic food doesn't go on sale much or have coupons, although I've noticed that has been changing over the past year, but the majority of coupons are for processed foods. Fruit sort of goes "on sale" when it's in season.

Shopping with Children

I went to the beach with a group of local moms, and of course, we started talking about food. The topic naturally diverged into a discussion about grocery shopping. One mom, Kate, said with her British accent, "I order my groceries and products online with Safeway every week, have them delivered, and the fee is only six dollars. I'm really happy with the quality of the food and the store is great about handling any complaints." My mouth hung open: "What! I spend endless amounts of time shopping for food! How is this possible?" I told my friend Jennifer about this phenomenon.

Jennifer did it for a while when she had her second baby and absolutely loved it, too. She said it saved her sanity and explained to me that you have to spend a certain amount of money, I think over $100.00, to get the cheap delivery rate. Many of us also have few relatives around to help and having a mother's helper doesn't come cheap or easily these days. When we're not in the throes of raising our little ones, we forget how intense and demanding parenting can be. After Jennifer's baby became a toddler and things weren't so intense, Jennifer quit ordering online because she found that she wanted to pick her own food. Food shopping with small kids isn't easy. There are other bonuses to this online shopping style. Children don't have to be exposed to all the Dora and Diego toys and candy bins when physically going into a regular grocery store.

While visiting my parents, I went to a large Fiesta store in Wisconsin, and they had a drop-in childcare play room for kids while parents shopped. I could see it as a great service for many parents. Sometimes we end up feeding our kids some kind of baked goods, crackers, or sweets while they sit in the grocery cart, too, just so we can get through the store without getting kicked out. A local parent told me his child really did get banned from the neighborhood health food store for unruly behavior. It seems that this service is really great, if it's available in one's area, for overwhelmed parents with young children.

I'm pleased with my shopping experience at my local health food store, New Leaf, because there is a level of community, support, and knowledge available there that is not found at a large corporate grocery store. And my experience with New Leaf's cashiers is different than at other stores, much more personal.

One of New Leaf's cashiers, Jill, raised three children of her own. She's still very attractive in her sixties, and no doubt must have been drop dead gorgeous in her twenties. She knew me when I waddled through her checkout line pregnant. She would always greet with a sweet and cheerful "Hello, Honey!" When she got a chance to see baby Savanah in my arms, she said, sweet and cheerful as ever, "Honey, if you ever need a babysitter, I'll take care of Savanah." I took her up on that, and to this day, Savanah adores this woman to no end. Savanah quivers with delight whenever she utters her name, "Jill," as if Jill were a big piece of candy. Jill is such a darling, kind-hearted person that she comes to Savanah's special events, everything from dance performances to birthday parties, just like a second mom or aunt.

Cashiers are well recognized in my community. Chris is another interesting one at New Leaf. He's always got the same down-key greeting, "Hi, how ya doin'? Hi, Savanah." He's an older bachelor, no kids, who volunteers much of his free time at the Wildlife Rescue Center. Savanah loves most of these cashiers and wants to show them anything new she has in her hands or tell them something she's doing. Michael, my husband, suggested once that the New Leaf staff was much more "real," and I agreed. They are real, even charmingly so. New Leaf is a small, but growing, community market chain, and at its current size, it is easier to get acquainted with like-minded health achievers and people concerned with better feeding, and naturally, you run into people like Chris who are also devoted to the health of the planet.

I read "The Three Bears" to Savanah, and porridge came up a fair amount, much like it did in the rhyme, "Peas porridge hot, peas porridge cold..." I started wondering what people used to eat and what they meant by "porridge." One day I asked Cindy, the 57-year-old, raven haired Italian beauty who maintains the bulk section at New Leaf: "What whole grain does rolled oats, oatmeal, come from?" She said, "Oat groats," and pointed to the bin. She added, "They take a little longer to cook." I used to cook oat groats but gave up on them. I just don't enjoy them as much as the faster cooking rolled oats.

But I buy all my grains from the bulk bins. My neighbor and mom friend, Hilde, said, "I priced the difference between the packaged oatmeal from Trader Joe's and the bulk oatmeal at New Leaf, and it's cheaper to buy it at New Leaf." These are the kind of head-scratching word problems to teach in Math: *If*, let's say, *12 oz. of organic oatmeal sells at Trader Joe's for $2.99 and organic rolled oats are $1.90 per pound at New Leaf, which one is the better deal?* I appreciated Hilde's help with the math.

In the end, I go to eight to ten different places to shop for food every season, and I buy specialty products online sometimes, like organic, raw nuts and olives, or green powders, because I read nuts can go rancid in the bulk bins. No one can say I don't shop for food. Still I can't brag that I'm a savvy shopper.

Savanah has done a lot of food shopping with me, and I wonder what all this shopping for food is doing to her. Once when she wasn't well and all she could do was lie around, she asked, "Daddy, will you carry me around New Leaf, and we can look at stuff." And he did. I thought that was interesting. Is it a comforting place for her? New Leaf does smell clean, and I know Savanah smells everything just like my childhood friend, Linda, did. I'm too afraid to smell everything. For example, at New Leaf the natural detergent and cleaning section passes by almost unnoticed. At a regular, commercial store, because the combined odors of the dyes and perfumes are so caustic, I hold my breath, run down to the detergent area to check to see if the unscented natural laundry soap is on sale and run back out. Despite her little nose, Savanah also possesses a knowledge of peoples' individual scents. Once her friend, Alana, left her slightly worn little girl white sandals that were the identical brand and size as Savanah's. "Which ones are yours, Savanah?" I asked her. She picked one up, smelled it, and pronounced: "These are Alana's." Maybe that's what all this food shopping has done, given Savanah an acute smelling ability.

Before the economic downturn, I used to simply go to the health food store and the farmers market. I considered the insanity around all my shopping and mediocre shopping skills. I talked with another mom who has three kids while we waited outside the classroom to pick up our kindergarteners. I told her, "I've been thinking about how much food shopping I'm doing. It's pretty crazy, all the places I go. How 'bout you? Do you go a lot of places?" Swiftly, she said, "No, not really. I just go to New Leaf and the farmers market; sometimes I'll stop in Safeway during the week." I probed her further, "Do you ever go to Trader Joe's?" She recalled, "Oh, yes, I go there for the non-dairy items. It's much cheaper." Then she began to relating another story about how she was with the kids at yet another grocery store, and in the middle of it, she stopped and smiled, "I guess my shopping is pretty crazy, too."

Most parents are on a budget. What a distraction all this shopping is and what a way to live life. I understand some people just go to Wal-Mart or Sam's Club, two other mega chain stores like Costco, and buy everything there on Saturday and fill up two grocery carts, while perhaps running to the store once during the week for some milk. I can't go to Wal-Mart, because for one, it's an hour's drive from my house, and, two, my mother follows the news. She once told me, "Wal-Mart doesn't treat their employees well. I don't like to shop there." Once you get into the mindset of considering every purchase you make as a vote, you start getting into the complex learning process of figuring out where food comes from, how employees are treated, which companies are doing things that are healthy and beneficial for others and the planet, such as donating a percentage of their profit to their local schools or encouraging consumers to go green by using less plastic bags and more biodegradable ones. This learning process can also be a tall order for tired parents.

The Farmers Market

I enjoy going to farmers markets. Savanah's gone to farmers markets quite a bit, and these outings have connected her to whole foods and learning what foods are ripe during the different seasons. Most stores do give a good idea of what is in season, but it's easiest to tell when visiting farmers markets. Kids love, need, thrive, and are guided by color, and the farmers markets give a lovely color show for children, colors they might not see otherwise after things are processed and cooked.

Rainbows, sunshine, and color, light energy, and vibrations are said to nourish our eyes, our bodies, and our souls. This year Savanah is five, and now she lives for the weekly neon, rainbow colored shaved ice at the farmers market. It's a miracle she made it to age five before I gave into the shaved ice. One reason why it took so long is that I went more often to a farmers market that keeps the baked goodies and other vendors in a separate aisle and section away from the farmers (yay, Aptos, CA farmers market!).

But recently, for something to do, I've been taking Savanah to one right down the street from us regularly, and I'm flat broke on cleverness. I just can't say no to her when all the other kids are so happy with their artificial blood red, lemon, and blueberry mounds of shaved ice. I bought time for a while by letting Savanah choose fresh cut flowers instead of shaved ice. Necessity being the mother of invention, we also made up our own sweetened strawberry slush recipe at home as a substitute, and it bought me some more time. Savanah wouldn't even have birthday cake at a party, if given the choice between the cake and shaved ice. It's too bad that the markets feel they have to allow junk food stands to attract customers. Once something like that is introduced, it's hard to get rid of. It wasn't that long ago that farmers markets never had other foodstuff except garden crops.

Color nourishes us and on levels we can't fully comprehend. In the past few years, phytonutrients have emerged in the science of nutrition and play a big role in new skin care products as well. Experts talk about phytonutrients with a mild-level ecstasy.

Phytonutrients are plant nutrients found in the colors of natural fruits and vegetables. They are touted for having remarkable healing benefits, warding off diseases, and promoting optimal health. What if we thought about our child's nutrition in terms of what color foods they ate each day? Some people do.

Savanah once noticed tangerines in season. "Mama," she said, "let's bring those small orange balls home." She ate three, four, seven of them in one sitting. "These are too good, Mama," she squealed. We once planned our next day's menu by color: "Let's see, purple cabbage, yellow squash, brown rice, orange carrots, green celery and red strawberries." We can engage our children in shopping for healthier foods by transforming shopping into a color treasure hunt. "Find something green, red, and purple." Our children will get to learn names and connect seasons with produce, and maybe their health benefits.

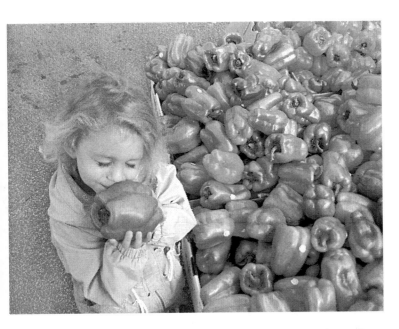

Savanah smelling the red peppers at the Aptos, CA farmers market.

Whenever I travel, I try to stop at local farmers markets. I've noticed that we've got a pretty good kids' section going on at the one down my street that functions a lot like the childcare play center at the Fiesta store in my parents' home town, while I've been to others that don't have kids' sections at all. Kid areas are great because it allows parents to shop more and spend money, while their kids play with other kids. My Felton Market is overseen by a board. This year, they improved the children's section by putting up a tent, and under the tent were tables with chairs, a children's play area with a green turf rug that housed the same dirty, old plastic Lego blocks and dinosaur figurines used year to year, which, amazingly, the kids never tire of. One table was covered with a paper table cloth and miscellaneous crayons were strewn on it, and this attracted many to coloring. Savanah and I went regularly this year just to hang out and talk with other parents.

The Garden

The dump truck quickly backed into our drive way, dumped a heap of black soil, and drove off. Fortunately, Michael had thought to purchase a large sheet of plastic, which we laid on our driveway so that we could get all the dirt to our new garden boxes, and not leave a dirty mess. Michael handed me a shovel. We began digging the dirt up into a wheel barrow. After the first load, I gripped the wheelbarrow handles to lift up a hulking mound of dirt over to the not-so-far-away garden box that Michael had built out of redwood. I couldn't budge the wheelbarrow with all its weight. I stepped aside for Michael. During the next filling of the wheelbarrow load, Michael stopped me. "You're going to hurt your back if you keep shoveling that way," he said. My back was hurting two minutes into the work. He was right. He demonstrated ergonomic shoveling, and I *tried* to copy his example, but I could still feel that I didn't get it. I dream of having three acres of land, but to be practical, I have all I can do to learn, manage, grow food and take care of just my little garden and yard.

There's a powerful book series called *The Ringing Cedars of Russia*. One of the tenets of the text is a call to return to the land, and more specifically a call to families to return to their own motherland of two and half acres or more. Anastasia, the main character, also encourages people to begin where they are—even planting and caring for one simple plant is a step in the right direction. I marvel at the visions put forth in these sacred texts. I am not a native Californian either, so I am learning the flowers and fruits of the seasons. Savanah and I do this together. I want Savanah to be skilled enough to cultivate her own motherland if she chooses to do so. As these books illustrate well, we've lost so much of our knowledge about plants, growing, and seasons. At the same time, I am definitely seeing a huge interest and effort in my greater community with giving kids experience by letting them play with nature, agriculture, and environmental events.

Learning about gardening is an endeavor of a lifetime, an endless, bountiful process that is good for adults as well as children. I believe the garden is truly the answer as the source of health and wisdom for our children and the planet. Having a garden and eating our own food is the least controversial health subject and receives worldwide affirmation. Most agree growing food is right on. Our culture is fiercely distracted with homework, lessons, computers, birthday parties, or the worst of circumstances, living in one of the ubiquitous endangered human habitats—homes surrounded by man made structures, cement and little in the way of nature's grass, trees, and food growing opportunities. Many things are important in the wellbeing of children, but as I continue to ponder the needs of feeding them, I am convinced that nothing is more essential than a garden.

One of the hallmarks of the popular Montessori education method is bringing daily life to the child's level. For example, a Montessori school may have light switches, sinks and counters at a child's height in order to allow children to do what they naturally want to do and that is: to do things themselves. My little two-year-old friend, Juliette, puts on her own shoes or pulls off her own cucumber from our garden she says, "I did it." About the same age as Juliette, I bought Savanah some child-sized gardening tools, including a cutter and hand shovels from a Montessori vendor. The quality of these gardening tools is so nice that sometimes I prefer to work with 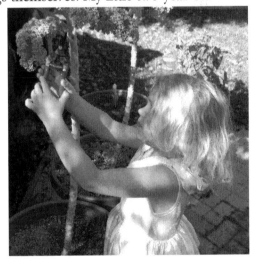 Savanah's garden tools over mine, which says it's time to get myself some new ones. The garden pots and boxes might be even more inviting for children because they are at the child's eye and hand level as opposed to rows of plants on the ground.

Pictured on the following page is Savanah, sticking her face into a Red Russian kale. It's rare to have a child who eats raw kale at the dinner table. I'm amused and elated as I watch her nibbling from the garden. One of her regular snacks includes parsley. It grows year 'round in our garden like a weed. I used to listen with delighted suspicion to her frequent confessions of devotion for this bitter herb. Many times I see her little friends join in with her for fun and stuff parsley in their mouths just because Savanah loves to do it.

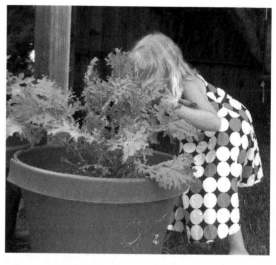

Her younger three-year-old friend, Kalani, came over once and had parsley from our garden and her mother says Kalani now insists that she pack parsley daily for lunch at preschool. Another day her good-for-getting-silly-with friend, Gillian, was over, and the both of them pulled off pieces of broccoli leaves and gobbled them down just for kicks and giggles. My niece, a regular white bread and sugar eater, happily nibbled daily from the garden when she visited last, which tells me that if kids have access they will eat garden foods. It feels good to offer a positive influence. The only problem is I have to get better at marking and remembering what herbs I planted. The kids ask, "What herb is this?" "Heck, I don't know," I say.

When Savanah was three or so I watched her joyfully dart around the garden. She'd stop at each plant, flutter her fingers in the leaves, and say, "Hi, kale! Hi, peas! Hi, cucumber!" Talking to trees and plants is a great way to cut yourself loose from the stressful, synthetic routine of the day; it connects you to the natural pulse of the earth, and it's also very good for the plants because they thrive off carbon dioxide. Stress management books also recommend gardening as concrete action for managing daily stresses. Even the smallest efforts of planting and beginning a garden are not insignificant. Watching food grow is fun! As soon as a broccoli floweret or a rose bud appears that we planted together, Savanah announces the new birth like a discovery, or as if she is on a treasure hunt in the yard. I am surprised at how eagle-eyed and in tune with the garden she can be. For people who only have room to plant a large pot or two, I recommend peas, cucumbers and tomatoes because they are very popular with kids. Children consistently come over and love to cut their own cucumber from the plant and pick the tomatoes and peas.

Giving Children More Access

In my area, a lot of families aren't able to have gardens because we live among the tallest trees on earth, the majestic Redwoods. Others just don't have the time, interest, or resources for gardening. Instead, many join a Community Supported Agriculture (CSA) farm coop and pick up their weekly box of fresh, locally grown, seasonal produce. Another option we have is to enroll our children in a summer program or school that exposes them to gardens. Many people are working to support school field trips to apple orchards, farms, and botanical gardens. It's another way we can get more kids connected to foods from the earth. Early childhood exposure to gardens is truly important for our children. Given the health crisis of our nation's kids, it's a priority. One in five children in the United States is overweight and 10% are classified as obese. Also plaguing our society are juvenile diabetes, early childhood tooth decay, food allergies, attention deficit hyper activity, autism and more.

I recall the summer vegetables and strawberry garden in my backyard as a child. "Can't go swimming until those strawberries are picked," mom reminded us from the back door. What stands foremost in my mind is that I was responsible for watering the house plants all year long. I simply watered each plant well once a week. I experienced the success of thriving house plants. I did feel connected and responsible for those house plants. I would have felt bad if they died, and I took pride in seeing them flourish. It's often challenging to find real work to assign our small children who want to help around the house and older kids who need to pitch in. I give two green thumbs up for delegating watering house plants to the kiddos.

School gardens are quickly gaining popularity. In our school lunch effort, Deidre and I visited the garden at our local public elementary school. The garden teacher began her class that day by offering

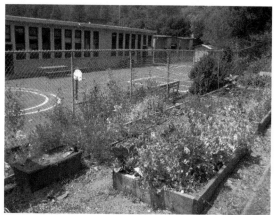

freshly pulled carrots from the school's garden to the energetic kindergarteners. Most of the kids learned for the first time what carrots look like coming from the ground. Except for one uninterested child, they each ate their little raw carrot off of its green top. Next, the kids all gathered to see and take a green bean upstart. They each got a small hand shovel, dug a hole, placed their bean plant in the ground and watered it. Afterwards, we talked with the teacher. We learned that the teacher worked part-time and that the garden was otherwise completely funded by the elementary school's parent group, the Parent-Teacher Association. The garden program existed year to year based on this support. In order to carry out the lesson and while ten children attended the garden activities, other parents volunteered along with one working staff to watch the rest of the class play on the playground and then they rotated the kids. The kids had to line up a couple of times, and wait for everyone to be on task together in order for things to go safely and smoothly in the garden. Although certainly the garden program is advantageous, I am glad that Savanah has the freedom to romp in her own garden, to pull leaves and flower petals and throw them up in the air, or to pick and eat the food at will.

The garden is our enduring teacher and friend. She trains our children effortlessly. Through her, our children are nourished and can experience a heightened sensitivity to the seasons and natural rhythms of growth and harvest. The garden provides children with the right foods to eat, and teaches them how to be well and to live a longer, healthier life. An organic garden gives a parent, who's adamant about feeding their child well, a distinct advantage.

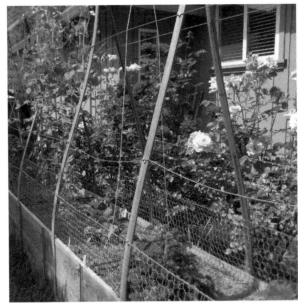

After five years of growing food in pots and garden boxes, there are two things that stand out in my mind this fall season. One, we get close to 100% of food we plant because it is in a controlled environment, meaning the food is not only in the garden boxes but netting is in the bottom around the top sides so that the moles and other animals can't get to it.

Shumei reports that about one-third of natural farm gardening is given over to nature, so the actual amount of food we can grow from our yard is actually quite significant. The other thing this year is that we stopped all planting at the end of the summer season and spent a weekend reworking the front yard garden box to break up the soil. We went through every inch, mostly by hand, and we discarded a lot of old plant roots. Every year we add and mix in a new top layer of organic soil and fertilizer, one being bat fertilizer. I wonder how bat poop gets collected. Savanah complained, "This day isn't fun. All we're doing is working." I do find the whole gardening thing to be a significant amount of work and some money. I also find it to be a source of sanity, inspiration, and comfort.

Less Meat

I live in a highly vegetarian-minded community, and yet, it seems that many of our families feed their children meat. In some cases, the parents may maintain a strictly vegetarian diet but will still feed their children meat. This is understandable. It's challenging enough just to feed children, period. Adding *any* restrictions just makes feeding our children nearly impossible. When I sat down to address better feeding in my writing, a meat diet was one of my foremost concerns: its high cost, the treatment of animals before and during death, antibiotics used on them, the effects of mass meat production on our planet, what it's doing to the American diet, especially in children.

Proponents of meat diets stress moderation; it is harrowing to see our children stuff themselves on *any* type of food, and even worse, to watch them gorge themselves on highly processed meat like chicken nuggets, hot dogs, lunch meats, fast food burgers. A contributing writer of E-How suggests that children ages two to three get 1,000 to 1,400 calories a day[1]. If a child with a sedentary lifestyle eats four pieces of McDonald's McNuggets, he or she is already pumping 170-190 calories[2] into his or her body, at 2.3 ounces that may or may not keep our children full for one whole meal. There are some exceptions featured in this book, like Pam's child, who can't eat almost anything without vomiting or breaking out into hives *except* for McDonald's food.

It is difficult not to envision certain foods as morally "evil" or "bad," but I persist for the sake of exceptions in every person's diet. Every family's lifestyle hosts new challenges. One mother in my community is a vegetarian, while the father and the kids aren't, and

---

[1] http://www.ehow.com/about_5339712_many-calories-do-children-need.html; as seen from http://www.mayoclinic.com/health/nutrition-for-kids/NU00606 and http://www.americanheart.org/presenter.jhtml?identifier=3033999

[2] http://www.scribd.com/doc/222559/McDonalds-Nutrition-Facts (170 calories) or http://www.thedailyplate.com/nutrition-calories/food/mcdonalds (190 calories)

hey say it works out just fine. A few families I know try to buy local, fresh, humanely grown, or grass fed meats, but this kind of meat is still not common and is significantly more expensive. In a junk food society, mostly not eating meat has saved Savanah from a lot of chicken nuggets, hotdogs, and fast food burgers. I'm amazed that at six years of age, she still does not have the concept of McDonald's and we drive by fast food restaurants almost daily. I have my doubts that this will last much longer.

When Savanah began preschool, she was old enough to notice the dinosaur chicken nuggets and turkey sandwiches. The first time she was there, the teacher brought out lunch saying, "Here's a half of turkey sandwich for everyone. And the peanut butter one is for Savanah." Like most kids, Savanah didn't want to be left out. She asked, "Can I have a turkey sandwich?" I happened to be there and said, "Sure." She took one tiny bite of her first piece of meat, very quietly put it down, and didn't touch it again. She had never tasted anything like it before. I asked the teacher if she would sanction her lunch day, try something vegetarian on Savanah's behalf. The teacher was happy to comply, but she said, "I will need help on lunch ideas that all the kids will like eating because they're all meat eaters."

Savanah's teacher and I went through a series of trial of error. I brought tamales one day, and beans and rice another. Both failed. Her teacher made two different lentil dishes. These also failed. None of the kids were used to eating beans. I gave up on my preschool and let the teacher make whatever would work to feed the gang, and it was things like macaroni and cheese. I was just glad to have a break from thinking about feeding Savanah for two meals a week.

Another day at preschool, Savanah's teacher presented a raw turkey, and the kids made stuffing, and stuffed the turkey together. This was Savanah's first, literally hands-on experience with meat. The turkey legs were bound together. Savanah looked to her teacher and asked wishfully: "If we untie its legs, do you think it can come back to life again?"

Out of eleven local preschools and childcare facilities in my area that I looked into, only one serves vegetarian lunches. A few programs serve vegetarian snacks while the parents provide and send lunches for their child. Two other preschools have lentil dishes on their menu and must have some measure of success with them.

Once I confessed to my respected friend, Dennis. He is a distributor of health books, and has been contemplating and living natural health for over forty years. He turned sixty this year and has enjoyed good health his entire life. "Savanah eats a lot of beans and rice," I said, and I might have been cringing without knowing it. It's difficult to know what to feed her, and sometimes I'll settle for anything that works, even if it means a lack of variety in her diet. He responded, "There's nothing wrong with beans and rice." This was a great comfort to me. Dennis is someone who prioritizes daily to nourish himself, and he more than anyone would know what is okay for our bodies to eat. I also thought about how many kids are allergic to various foods—soy, dairy, nuts, eggs, and wheat, but I haven't heard any reports of issues around beans, but allergies are one thing, and getting kids to eat these beans are another

Our first few weeks at Natural Foods Wednesday at my local school district had some measure of success, but even when the black beans and rice lunch entrée was freshly-made and offered, the kids did not like it. For now, this entrée has been canceled. Although beans are a staple in Mexican cuisine, bean meals are not common in this country. I learned the basics about how to cook beans for optimal digestion from *Romancing the Bean: Essentials for Creating Vegetarian Bean Dishes* by Joanne Saltzman. It would be lovely if all these cooking shows currently on television showed us how to cook and prepare more vegetarian dishes. Every time I channel surf to one, the entrée is always meat. Our children and the planet will be more healthful if more families can become skilled at how to cook beans, and get their kids to eat more beans and rice.

Raising a child as a vegetarian is easier today. Around the 1940s, my old-timer friend, Arthur, said his mother didn't speak to him for years when he became a vegetarian because he wouldn't eat her food. Today, it is not uncommon to meet people who grew up as vegetarians or others who came from religious sects like the respected vegetarian diet of Seventh Day Adventists. One thing I know for sure is that too much strictness, too many rules, and too many no's around food back fires. In the previous chapter on sugar, I addressed some of the issues around both forbidding and allowing oo much of it, and the same rule of thumb applies for meat. In the beginning and still to some extent, our friends and family worried about what to feed us when we came. I always brought food, but as Savanah got older and started going to play for longer stretches at other people's homes, I introduced to her peanut butter and jelly sandwiches, because peanut butter and jelly sandwiches are something easy and most people have. It was interesting that she did not like peanut butter right away.

Restrictions

I went to a baby shower and met an older but youthful mom named Karen who had two boys, ages five and seven. As we touched upon the topic of feeding children in our conversation, I admired her clarity and her disciplined ability to stay true to whole foods for her family. She said her son got sick as a small child, and she was able to get her son well by changing the diet of the whole family. She followed a vegetarian, macrobiotic-whole foods diet. She did not feed or allow her kids any junk food. She seemed to exemplify what all the health books suggest. She said, "If we have something sweet like pumpkin pie, we make it ourselves." Karen taught me how to make and serve more whole grains like amaranth, oat groats, quinoa, and buckwheat (from the four, I came out using quinoa on fairly regular basis).

Sometime later, Karen and I were shopping at our local health food store and I walked around with her to see what products she used. While we did this, I noticed her boys begging for various sugary products. Each time the boys pleaded, Karen firmly said, "No." I commented on this: "They still keep asking after all this time of never buying the stuff, and you have to just keep saying no?" She nodded. "Yes, even when the answer is always no, they still beg." While we shopped, I noticed Karen's boys were strong and skinny, almost uncomfortably thin, for American standards. The boys ate three regular meals a day, no junk food, no snacking in between. She home-schooled her boys in the morning, and they got regular fresh air and hard exercise every afternoon. I've met up with her in the afternoons and watched the boys run and chase each other for hours down hiking paths through the forest and swim and play at the river.

Then, Karen's family went on an extended trip to Europe to meet up with her husband's side of the family. It's common that all our resolve to feed kids well can get thrown out the window with a single visit to grandma and grandpa's. It is precisely for this reason that I like to ask parents about food and dining during their travels or visits with relatives. I ran into Karen at the health food store, and it was one of the first things I mentioned. I thought casually about the reputation of the English for consuming lots of meat, and asked Karen, "So, how did the whole eating thing go while you were in Europe?" Karen said, "I'm almost embarrassed to show you this," and pointed to the lean, organic meats in her shopping basket. She said, "The boys ate meat at the relatives and loved it. I keep the red meat to once a week. I don't know how or what else to feed such hungry, growing boys. They eat much more than I do now." I nodded. As our children grow older, such as during ages nine to eighteen, it almost seems necessary to buy a dump truck to feed them, especially males leading an extremely physically active lifestyle. Even 3,200 calories might not be enough for their bodies, which can and do sprout like legendary bean stalks.

Roughly a year later, Karen found herself in a sudden, difficult, and complicated divorce. Her husband traveled a lot for his job and ended up meeting another woman. He fought for full custody of the boys. As part of the battle, Karen's husband got his family to write letters about the way she feeds, or perhaps, doesn't feed the children. Those letters were enough to force Karen through psychological testing and parent shadowing. She was literally accused of being a "health nut." During the custody battle, the boys got to eat whatever they wanted with their father: pizza, ice cream, and whatever else they were *deprived* of. In the end, they have shared custody. Karen continues to eat well and live by example for her boys, and the boys are also older now and make their own choices.

Quest for Meat

Books, discussions, and arguments over the pros and cons of eating a meat- or plant-based diet are nearly endless; however, the grave problems with the high meat consumption path that Americans have been on can no longer be ignored. Just a few of the significant works on this subject are the *U.N. Food and Agriculture Organization 2006 Report*, best-selling Pulitzer Prize winning book, *Diet for a New*

America by John Robbins, *The Omnivore's Dilemma* by Michael Pollan, Jane Goodall's book, *Harvest of Hope*, as well as documentary films like *Supersize Me* and *Food Inc.* As we've gained more understanding about the fattening and treatment of cows before slaughter with fossil fuel-based fertilized soybeans and corn, and the required antibiotics used in feeding them, it's harder to turn a blind eye to the quality and cost of this meat.

The *U.N. Food and Agriculture Organization 2006 Report* notes that conventional livestock raising is adding more greenhouse gas emissions to the planet than transportation.[3] The meat industry disputes this amount. Even if the report is not completely accurate, livestock emissions fall in line with serious issues like cars and air pollution. Moreover, the huge demand of corn for feeding our beef industry is depleting our soil resources in the U.S., and we continue to destroy vast amounts of rain forests to grow soybeans and corn to feed cows. In addition, the final cattle fattening in feedlots bolsters their unhealthy saturated fat content.

Another sobering fact is how cruel we actually treat animals commercially-raised for food. These animals endure unspeakable living conditions and force feedings to make them plump and get them to market sooner. There's a ghastly photo in Jane Goodall's book, *Harvest of Hope*, of a bird with a hose shoved down its throat enduring a force feed. Because of these woefully unhealthful conditions, antibiotics are necessary to be injected into the animals and often growth hormones are used as well.

Maybe children *do* need meat to grow stronger, healthier bodies. *Nourishing Traditions* is an influential book out now based on the work of Weston Price. This book describes how natural meats hardly exist today. Not that long ago, animals used to graze on green grasses filled with chlorophyll and other natural nutrients, and that nourishment was transferred to the consumer. Now the vast majority of animals raised for consumption are corn and grain fed.

In 2009, and inspired by *Nourishing Traditions*, I went out looking for chicken and beef bones for soup broth. I found it strange that I could not obtain chicken bones at the conventional or health food store meat departments. Amongst all the meat products, both

---

[3] TIME magazine, January 12, 2010

places had only a few packages of beef bones. The butcher at the commercial supermarket said all the meat comes precut and packaged now. Of the few beef bones, the butcher from the health food store said that bones came from cows that were corn fed. Of all the cuts of meat at the natural foods store, only two cuts were from grass fed cows.

I finally noticed the ranch with the grass fed meat booth at one of my local farmers markets. I asked for a soup bone with as little meat on it as possible, and the rancher told me the name of the bone, which failed to register anything in my brain. I grew up eating meat, my father has a degree in agricultural economics, and I have next to zero knowledge of cow anatomy. What's a shank bone? At home, I threw the nameless bone in the crock pot with water and vegetables and let it cook all day. As I served it for dinner, I saw small globs of meat fat floating on the soup's surface. I served a bowl to Savanah with a cheerful voice: "This is soup cooked with a cow bone, and it supposed to make your body and bones strong." She was caught off guard and slurped up a spoonful. "Yuck! I can't eat this stuff! Taste terrible! Do you like it?" I took a spoonful. It was wretched-tasting to me, too. No amount of bullion or sugar was going to cover up that taste. When you're not used to eating meat, it's very foreign-tasting and smelling, especially when it's not disguised with ketchup, mustard, and mayonnaise.

I also bought and cooked some grass fed beef twice a week for a few months to see if I could increase my low iron level and if Savanah might like it. I was informed that because grass fed beef is less fatty than commercially raised beef, it requires different cooking considerations and sometimes more chewing. Savanah did not like the smell of the meat in the house, and looked upon it with disdain as I ate. During this trial period, she never came around to taking a single bite. After a few months and another blood test, my iron level remained unchanged, and I imagine from all that I've read, I found little pleasure in eating meat and discontinued.

I have also since heard that Weston Price conclusions, the work behind *Nourishing Traditions,* have been discounted by many current doctors and are said to not have been based on scientifically sound research methods. When I read Weston Price, and all these health books for that matter, they are all very convincing. It's challenging and confusing for parents.

On another visit with my friends, Cecile, who learned to grow magnificent fruits and vegetable gardens in her fifties, and Dennis, our conversation, as always, turned to food and gardening, what fruit is in season now, or how their melons did this year. They live on five acres of land that mainly Cecile works year round. We talked about feeding kids. Dennis said, "I've never raised a child. I know it's hard, but I'm still saying what I've been saying for years: a low protein, low fat, high carb diet will cure many of our diseases. I always point to The China Study. That is the largest, most intensive, controlled health study ever conducted and probably ever will be, and that's exactly what came out of that study about health: Eat a low protein, low fat diet." Cecile added that Dr. Campbell discovered that he could turn cancer on and off by increasing and decreasing the amount of animal protein ingested, and concluded that human's need only 10% of their calories from protein and that plant protein was the most efficient source.

The China Study by Dr. Campbell, a professor of nutritional biochemistry at Cornell University, and his son, Thomas Campbell recommends that people should eat a whole food, plant-based diet and avoid consuming beef, poultry, and milk as a means to minimize and/or reverse the developments of chronic disease. *The China Study* also recommends that people should take in adequate amounts of sunshine in order to maintain sufficient levels of vitamin D and consider taking dietary supplements of vitamin B_{12}. Savanah gets a lot of outside activity, and I give her a supplement with B_{12}, but I can't help but wonder if it's enough. Dennis and Cecile also added that the following current and respected, western trained doctors and authors all pretty much agree that the best diet to eat to prevent all the major chronic diseases is a low-fat, low protein, plant based diet: Dr. McDougall, Dr. Fuhrman, Dr. Esselstyn, Dr. T. Colin Cambell and Dr. Ornish. Dr. Fuhrman has a book called *Disease Proof Your Kids*.

I shared with Dennis my concern about calcium and growing bones. Dennis responded, "It's a high protein diet that makes the body have to use more calcium. Look at all those countries with low protein diets. They don't have osteoporosis problems."

Cecile encourages me to call Kim, a mom I met at her place some years ago who is raising two children on a plant based diet and had since moved to Oregon near Klamath Lake, famous for its blue green algae. I called Kim and her oldest is now eight. We talked about how she keeps her kids well fed and satisfied. And she agreed, her biggest strategy is "Keeping the kids fed" so that they are never left to eating whatever unhealthy food might be available.

Kim gave me a basic rundown on her family's meals: For breakfast it's usually a thick smoothie of raw eggs, almonds, bananas, and frozen fruit like cherries, strawberries and blueberries. She said that holds them until lunch. Then at lunch they have a salad with avocado and sesame and flax ground up. For mid afternoon snack it's usually fruit and almonds. Dinner is salad and all kinds of steamed vegetables; potatoes are a staple. They keep dulse flakes and nori in shakers on the table as regular condiments. She said they do eat a lot of bananas like a crate a week as well as avocados.

Kim is homeschooling and basically living off the grid. Kim agreed that as far as diet and sending kids off to school it's really hard— "leaving them to the dogs," she said. Savanah loves going to school. I love her going to school. I've met a few homeschooling families that are doing really well by their children as far diets, but in my experience I've found that to be the exception rather than the norm.

On his death bed, I asked my friend Arthur, who made it in Paul Nison's book, *Interviews with Health Achievers*: "What about protein, Arthur?" He whispered loudly, "Don't worry about protein! What is protein? Lots of people worry about protein, and they don't even know what it is. All food has some protein." Still, the following is a list of all the no-meat, higher protein foods I could find. Nutritiondata.com is a good website for finding out how much protein is in various foods.

Protein List

- Vegetables
- Eggs, cheese, yogurt
- Some pastas and cereals
- Enriched rice, soy, and nut milks

- Whole grain breads and other whole grains like quinoa and rice
- Soybeans (tofu, miso, edamame) and soy nuts
- Beans (pinto, black, navy, lentils, etc.) and hummus (garbanzo beans, also known as chickpeas)
- Nuts and seeds (hazelnut [also known as filberts], almond, walnut, pecan, pumpkin) and nut butters
- Supplements
- Bee pollen
- Blue green algae and Spirulina
- Goji berry

Meat Alternatives

Meat alternatives prove challenging for parents, too. As mentioned, many children (and parents) have sensitivities and difficulty digesting dairy, tofu, soy, wheat gluten, and nuts. For example, there's a product called Tofurkey. It tastes and smells just like turkey and is high in protein. It's made from wheat gluten and soy beans making it an impossible alternative for many. And if a child can't eat nut butters or nuts and seeds, then it seems that eating freshly cooked, humanely raised meats is required, and acceptance that the child may not be able to be raised as a vegan or vegetarian is also necessary.

The Goji Berry

The Goji berry grows on an evergreen shrub found in temperate and subtropical regions of China, Mongolia, and the Himalayas in Tibet, looks like red raisins and has the texture of raisins.[4] For those that have never tried it, it has a mildly tangy taste, a little on the sweet and sour side. Scientific information about the virtues of Goji berries is astounding. Goji berries have been touted as one of the super foods of the world and are extremely nutrient dense. Despite all these benefits and more, I've found Goji berries are a hard sell for kids.

---

[4] http://altmedicine.about.com/od/completeazindex/a/goji.htm

When Savanah was two or three, Michael and I bulk ordered bags of the freshest Goji berries we could find online. I started feeding Savanah Goji berries when she was little, and I could get away with it. I fed them to her in their dried fruit state and cooked them in her oatmeal, but it was not long before Savanah refused to eat her oatmeal with Goji berries cooked in it. I got Savanah and her little friends to eat Goji berries here and there and off and on, but the final conclusion was that the kids didn't like them. At best, I might cook up some tea with them and sneak a little of the juice in a smoothie, but as Savanah is almost six now, it's harder to hide super foods like this in her meals.

A big problem I found with Goji berries is that because they're like raisins, they get stuck in the back of the teeth. I was at the dentist getting my teeth cleaned one day, and brought Savanah along when she was three years old. For fun, the hygienist took a picture of her teeth, and she had just been snacking on Goji berries while she was waiting for me. The hygienist and I saw the red little berries coating the tiny crevices of her back teeth. She warned me, "You've got to be careful with things like that, fruit leather, raisins, and the like. That stuff rots the teeth."

Quinoa

Whole grains are a cornerstone of the macrobiotic diet and also not something I ate much growing up. Some of the grains I've tried without much success yet are amaranth, buckwheat, and millet. I have yet to make tasty dishes despite all the great recipes I've tried. On the other hand, my big learning curve paid off when I got a grip on quinoa. Quinoa is new for a lot of us because it's been reintroduced after falling out of the diet somewhere along the way. The ancient Incas used quinoa. Quinoa is considered the super grain alternative to rice[5], has a balanced set of amino acids, meaning it's a high-quality protein. And, it's gluten-free, easy to digest and, my favorite part, cooks in twenty minutes. Quinoa gives a mother feeding a child a vegetarian diet some peace of mind. I've used quinoa as a breakfast, lunch, and dinner food as well as baked with

---

[5] *"Quinoa, The Supergrain Alternative to Rice"* in *Hinduism Today*. Kapaa: Nov 30, 1991. Vol. 13, Iss. 11; pg. 16

quinoa flour, recipes for quinoa abound on the Internet. If you're going to try Quinoa and haven't before, you can find it easily in the bulk section at health food stores. I have the stainless steel Miracle Rice Cooker and Steamer. It's in constant use. I make quinoa in this cooker and throw the same pot with leftovers into the refrigerator for use the next day.

Nuts and Seeds

Raw, unprocessed, unsalted nuts and seeds, like flax, almond, pumpkin or sesame seeds provide the greatest amount of nutrition. Almonds are a huge staple in California. L.J. Grauke writes in the *Encyclopedia of Food and Culture* that almond trees "are planted in irrigated orchard configurations with densities of up to one hundred thirty-four trees per acre," as opposed to other locations, like Majorca, where they are lucky if they yield fifty to seventy trees. Along the I-5 through Central California, rows and rows of beautiful, heavily fertilized almond trees flag in the wind, sometimes bright with yield, about 3,000 pounds per acre achieved. The only problem with almond consumption is the amount of pesticides used to protect the trees, because it is unusually high. Almonds must be eaten in moderation anyway because they are a concentrated source of energy, relatively high in fat.

Nut butters can be successful with kids. Peanut butter does not rank high on a quality foods list and because it is high in mold, but certainly peanut butter provides for some nutrition and works for kids (note: a common misconception about the peanut is that it is considered a "nut," but peanuts are actually legumes or beans). One day Savanah said, "Peanut butter and jelly sandwiches are good for you." I said they are okay, but peanut butter is high in fat, so it's not good to eat too much peanut butter."

Savanah ate flax seed crackers and cashew butter (lowest in oil content) regularly between the ages of two and three and then wasn't interested in nuts or nut butters for a year or two. Lately, she's been eating raw almonds, which is a good reminder for me not to give up on healthy foods, as kids can have their ebbs and flows. Again, I could get away with the raw nuts when she was younger, but at almost six now I've resorted to the salted or roasted pistachios nuts and pumpkin seeds, so she will eat them here and there. I also try to soak larger nuts like pecans. This way they are easier for the body to digest. One of the great things about pecans is that they're indigenous to North America, found in the well-drained alluvial soils of the Mississippi River and from tributaries in Illinois and Iowa south to the Gulf Coast of Louisiana, and even out in Texas. Isolated populations of pecans are found as far south as Oaxaca, Mexico. The indigenousness of certain foods becomes integral to other aspects of this book that address global pollution and industry; I whole-heartedly promote local and domestic produce, because it cuts down on a lot of unnecessary pollution and other things harmful to people and the planet.[6]

Eggs

I wish I would have introduced hard boiled eggs earlier with Savanah, because maybe she would like them more now. She eats them now only with agave ketchup poured over them. Eggs have gone in and out of favor over the years. Eggs are a whole food. Many report they are a perfect food, but they are out of the range of the vegan diet. If you buy eggs, I've learned that *cage free* is a key phrase for conscious egg buyers to look for, because "free range" can mean a chicken was let out of its cage momentarily. I envy the growing number of people I know who are raising chickens with their kids. They get to see baby chicks and eat fresh eggs. Everybody I know who has chickens loves having them, but like having any animal, they are a responsibility. Eggs are a nutrient dense, high protein, whole food and thus a great protein option for kids.

Digestion

Dennis also commented to me once that he thought the missing key to understanding health in its entirety was about digestion. Meat and nuts take the body hours to digest, while foodstuffs like fruit digests much more quickly. Although numerous health books bring up the importance of good digestion, Russell Mariani in his book, *Healing Digestive Illnesses* (a big problem for many of us), masterfully

---

[6] "Nuts" by L. J. Grauke from Encyclopedia of Food and Culture. Ed. Solomon H. Katz. Vol. 2. New York: Charles Scribner's Sons, 2003. p605-614.

ddresses the need and art of proper digestion. The Macrobiotic nd Ayurveda paths also thoroughly address ways towards better ligestion.

'rom a raw foods perspective, enzymes are a key concept in ligestion. In the 1930s, after the discovery of vitamins and ninerals, enzymes were identified. Enzymes are present in raw 'oods, and they initiate the process of digestion in the mouth and tomach. The enzymes in raw food help start the process of ligestion and reduce the body's need to produce digestive enzymes. Raw food evangelist, David Wolfe, writes that "the discovery of ـnzymes is one of the greatest breakthroughs ever achieved in ١utrition." Only raw foods and enzyme supplements contain ـnzymes. Enzymes are destroyed by the cooking process. Enzymes ١elp with weight loss, accelerate detoxification/cleansing, and ؤreatly assist the digestive process. They transform amino acids, ًats, starches, and minerals. Enzymes also increase nutrient ٔssimilation and help rejuvenate aged skin and internal organs.[7]

In *Nourishing Traditions*, Sally Fallon writes that all enzymes "are deactivated at a wet-heat temperature of 118 degrees Fahrenheit and a dry-heat temperature of about 150 degrees." Food can still be warmed up and not lose all its natural enzymes. If food can be touched without pain (liquids over 118 degrees will burn), we can determine ourselves whether or not the food we are eating still contains its enzyme content.[8] Eating enzyme rich foods gives more energy because the body does not have to work so hard making its own enzymes to digest the food. I've come to understand that although bread, muffins, cookies, crackers, and other baked goods practically melt in our mouths and are so easy for us to eat, the body, however, has a hard time digesting them.

In *The Science and Fine Art of Food and Nutrition*, Herbert Shelton writes that our children "should be taught early to thoroughly masticate (chew) all food. This is best done by giving the child foods that require chewing when he or she first begins to eat solid food." He continues, "Many feed their children mushes and foods

[7] http://www.sunfood.com/Catalog/Default.aspx?gclid=CJ3DodzWlJ8CFR4Eagod-gqfmQ

[8] P.46, Sally Fallon, *Nourishing Traditions*

that have been put through a sieve, which may be swallowed without chewing. The result is they never learn to chew. If the child can't chew his or her food, he or she is not ready for that kind of food. Digestion begins in the mouth, children will develop a habit of not chewing and just swallowing food if they are given food that doesn't require chewing." [9] In *The Macrobiotic Path to Total Health*, Michio Kushi adds, "Thorough chewing is essential to digestion, and it is recommended that each mouthful of food be chewed fifty times or more until it becomes liquid in the mouth." [10]

The fine art of chewing is mostly ignored by the American culture; an average eat-in at McDonald's, for instance, takes 7 to 10 minutes, and even a group of five or six are asked to finish everything in 30 minutes. Most processed foods that you find in the "refrigerated" aisle of the grocery store are bite-sized, which encourages persons to literally swallow down as many pieces of pizza or other foods. While I eat with Savanah, sometimes I'll remember to play a chew-your-food game with her. So far she can get up to twenty chews, but her average has been twelve. I am aware of how poorly I chew my food, and, like so many other parents, I sometimes eat while I drive, a habit I try to avoid. I want to set a better example. As Mariani said, *how* we eat is just as important as what we eat.

Jane Goodall wrote eating less meat is the most effective contribution we can make to the health of the planet, but what does eating less meat look like or mean? On average, I would say American kids are eating meat once or twice a day. Kids might have a turkey or a peanut butter sandwich for lunch and a hamburger or chicken for dinner. How much less could kids and families eat each week and still feel and grow at their optimum?

There are numerous diet plans out there that prescribe how many ounces of protein to eat at each meal. I bought an inexpensive little digital scale years ago, and it continues to work great. I disciplined myself to weigh and measure food, and have found it useful in seeing what are considered "normal" proportions. In general, for adults the protein suggested per meal is between 3 and 6 ounces with 6 ounces being on the high end. I checked the school's

---

[9] P. 566-7, Herbert Shelton, *The Science and Fine Art of Food and Nutrition*

[10] P. 13, The Macrobiotic Path to Total Health, Michio Kushi

districts protein requirements for children. It ranges between 1.5 ounces to 3 ounces of protein, and in general my district sticks to 2 ounces of protein for all its school lunches. We are a nation whose one favorite past time is barbequing, and every barbeque I've ever gone to the meat servings far surpass 6 ounces. It may be useful to a parent on a budget or dealing with weight problems in the family, to get a scale and get a clear idea of how much protein they're serving at meals.

I've also weighed and measured nuts. Nuts are high in protein but they are also high in fat, too. I've found that I can't sit down and eat more 2 ounces of nuts at a time and eat all my vegetables and other foods at a meal. Nut protein weight is different than meat or dairy. 5 ounces of nuts would definitely be excessive and hard for the body to digest.

One mom friend, Lea, says her family's eating less meat because it's too expensive for the four of them. She says, "I really have to stretch the meat out. Like, when I make spaghetti or fajitas, everybody gets a little meat with their dinner. We eat a lot of peanut butter and jelly."

There are a number of books and studies out now that describe the benefits to the planet by even just eating one less meat meal a week. Some schools are doing Meatless Mondays for school lunches and cutting back on meat this way. Many health experts suggest that we don't all have to become vegetarian. We just need to cut back on the amount of meat and meat products we eat.[11] My friend, Mara, at age seventy and after thirty years of being a vegetarian started eating a little meat again, twice a week, enjoys it, and feels better. We don't have to be attached to these labels of "vegan," "meat eater" or "vegetarian." Our diets change as needed, but it is clear that that as a nation we need to learn how to consume less meat.

I make no claims of great success on this no-meat diet. We do eat *a lot* of beans and rice, usually one meal every day. In good times and in hard times, beans are what we eat. When we're on the run, it's a bean burrito. Savanah eats too many bean burritos and peanut butter and jelly sandwiches. I've got three staple beans I rotate on:

11 http://www.telegraph.co.uk/health/healthnews/6653675/Eat-less-meat-to-reduce-climate-change-and-save-thousands-of-lives.html

pinto, black, and lentil beans. My goal is to expand my bean repertoire. My approach to making most of bean dishes is very simple—some kind of bean in the crock pot with a little bullion, and Celtic salt. I make variations from there. I might add potatoes, onion, garlic, celery or carrots. This past summer, Savanah was tired of my bean dishes and wasn't in the mood for them during this hot season. I was thrown in a loop. "Okay kid, what are you going to eat besides some fruit and vegetables from the garden?"

I've tried cooking with and have eaten a little tofu and tempeh off and on for years, but I have never enjoyed much success with it. Sometimes people assume tofu (soybeans) are all vegetarians eat, but I have not found that to be the case for myself or with my friends who also eat a plant-based diet. Savanah has eaten a little of it here and there. I'm not big on feeding her a lot of dairy either, but she eats that off and on, too. Cheese, like peanut butter, is the common American alternative for meat at school.

Nothing works every time and change is certain. Sometimes she likes to eat nuts, often she doesn't. Quinoa is in one day and out the other. I continue to be challenged by this protein issue. I am not so much worried about the protein. As Arthur said, it's in everything. I am just trying to feed her meals so that she's satisfied and not hungry one hour later. Just last night at 8 p.m., when it was time for bed and stories, Savanah called out, "I'm still hungry!" I fell on the bed, looked up at the ceiling and hollered back to a little five-year-old, "Go in the kitchen and find something. I don't know what to feed you."

Concluding Thoughts

My hope is simply that this work helps--teachers, guardians, future parents, or those just wanting to live well. I want to accelerate our understanding on how to feed children well and help many of us figure out how to feed ourselves well, too. I want to encourage. Choosing a healthy lifestyle takes a tremendous amount of courage. I also want to bring closure to all the research, interviews, and experiences I have had up until now about vegetarian, low meat diets, and shed some light on what's been going on with school lunch.

It's funny. After all my research and experiences, I still have a challenge making a day's food plan. Every day Savanah comes to me multiple times, saying, "I'm hungry!" I argue back: "We just had lunch twenty minutes ago. You didn't eat enough. What do you want? " I make some suggestions. "Do you want an orange?" "No," she says. "Do you want an apple with some peanut butter?" I suggest further. "No," she says again. I'm doing a lot of shopping, preparing, putting food out, cleaning up, or thinking about what to have next for her and any other kids around. I ask myself, "With kids, can we go two hours without eating?"

Sometimes, more than technique, you have to have drive, tenacity, will power. If you understand inside of yourself that the body needs time to rest and digest and live a life apart from eating, you can supplement this. From my experience with sugar and Savanah's teeth, I have learned that you have to persist with feeding your child well even when they reject it, and say "no" when it isn't the appropriate time to eat, even if they feel hungry.

I am now basically doing what the school lunch program and other diet plans promote. I think of lunch and dinner as, *what do I have for a protein, starch, and vegetable,* so that I know she can be satisfied for a while and get more complete nutrition. At lunch and dinner, I ask her just like a food promoter, "What vegetable are you going to have?"

And she *has to eat one*. There's not going to be any treat or more of something unless she has some vegetables, and sometimes she does say, "How many more bites do I have to eat?"

Although recently I took my daughter and her friend, Natasha, to the local health food store to shop for their dinner. They wanted to make the soup and declared that it had to be healthy. They chose a box of organic, low sodium broth and then went to the produce section. Excitedly they bounced up and down the aisle saying out loud what they wanted to put in the soup. "Let's put kale and celery in it! Mom, can we put radishes in our soup?" Behind me came an older woman's voice in my ear that asked, "Where did you pick these kids up? Whoever heard of a kid liking radishes?"

We brought the goods home and the girls tore and cut vegetables with dull knives and dropped the variety into the pot. Fifteen minutes later we all sat down to eat their soup. The vegetables were undercooked and the soup was bland. Savanah and Natasha seem to be savoring each bite. I asked them, "How is your soup?" They smiled knowingly at each other and said in unison, "The best soup ever!"

I still shop three times a week to make sure I have fresh celery, tomatoes, snap peas, carrots, red peppers, cucumbers or cabbage, so I know I'll have something that appeals to her. I also do my best everyday to keep a container of vegetables in her school bag, in the car, and at the park, or where ever we go because she gets hungry. When that's what's readily available and crunchy, she eats it. And, unlike cooked foods, raw vegetables can sit out for hours without having to be refrigerated.

During the first month of Savanah's new school year, I was able to arrange a meeting for SLV LOCALS, our whole lunch, school garden, farm-to-school effort with the high school assistant principal, the nutrition director, Chef Kathy, Tim, Deidre, and myself. The assistant principal readily came on board with us, and approved Kimberly to work with the freshman Health class. Ninth graders are going to be given the opportunity to earn health credits working with nutrition services and with us to have a Health Expo for the younger students. The assistant principal said that "the health teacher is always ooking for good student projects, and this is a project that many kids oday are truly interested in." I left the meeting feeling very thrilled.

Meanwhile, it is clear that although we've successfully brought in ome organic, local and fresh veggies one day a week, the kids aren't eally eating them, and one reason is there's not enough staff to ncourage or help serve them the veggies. The old saying fits here: you can bring a horse to water but you can't make 'em drink." So far we've got a couple LOCAL parent volunteers to step in sometimes on our Natural Foods Wednesday and act as "Veggie Encouragers." Tim's pretty wife, Cheryl, was the first to step in. She posted to our SLV LOCALS Yahoo! group:

> "[I'm] happy to report that I really feel like I made a difference! I definitely encouraged many children that were skipping the veggies to take either a salad or a veggie side to go with their entree. A couple of kids didn't realize they could take a salad. Some just wanted help fitting the salad on their tray. Some just needed to hear 'crispy crunchy delicious... Goes great with your warm pasta!'

> "The kids *love* the carrots with the greens on them. They went fast! The bagged carrots, I noticed, didn't seem as popular. Reminding the kids with an enthusiastic voice and smile that the produce was grown locally did motivate a bunch of kids."

This simple smile and encouragement was the essence of my friend Arthur's career, along with great advice about dieting, exercise, overall health. He often said that positive thoughts are the food for the mind and soul and are even more important than the food we eat. Whenever I asked him if there was anything I could bring him or do for him, he always answered, "a smile and a kind word."

Joni, another mom in the SLVLOCALS group, stepped up for our other elementary school. I admire Joni. She's very sweet and willing to do service. She's a surfer, awesome with yarns and crafty projects with kids, travels to New Zealand every year for a holiday, and is a natural beauty in her forties. Joni wrote:

> "[I] just want to let you all know what a satisfying experience I had yesterday doing 'veggie pushing.' I'd say I got nearly

90% of the kids to get something from the veggie cart. My observations:

"#1 It works! The kids will take it if you offer. Kids have the habit of just going straight from the main food line to the cashier to pay, completely bypassing the veggie cart. I greeted each kid individually with a giant cheerful smile and asked them, 'Would you like a fresh carrot, or cucumber slice?—Some salad, or a little tomato, or broccoli with ranch dressing?'

It felt good to see the kids actually thinking about what they wanted. I consider that good training in tuning into their bodies. There were certainly some that just said, 'No, I'm good,' but very few in comparison to those who actually took something. And I'm certain that the kids who took the veggies ate theirs because it was a conscious choice they were making. They had decided themselves that the veggie they took sounded good to them that day.

"#2 There wasn't enough! I felt terrible about the fact that I had a paltry amount to give the children. I could have given out way more if there had been more. At the same time, I can understand that if no one had been there to push the veggies and the kids normally walk by it, what was there would have gone to waste.

"#3 A server is really important because of the physical challenge of getting the food. The children walk through the line holding a little cardboard box that gets filled up with their main menu item, drink, and utensils. By the time they get to the veggie cart, it's a huge challenge to juggle that and try to get a veggie container put together and in the box without help. It's hard to fit one more thing into their little lunch carrier things, and it's also challenging to get the vegetables out of their serving bowls (under the sneeze guard) with the plastic tongs.

"#4 Please, oh, please, can we get a core group to take turns doing this? It would be really fantastic to get a volunteer calendar going so that we had a parent there every Wednesday. It really didn't feel like a big time commitment for me, and it was probably the most satisfying hour I've spent in a long time feeling like I was really having an impact and making the kids happy. They just light up to get that kind of attention beamed at them, and I like that they can associate vegetables with a friendly interaction."

Unfortunately, ongoing volunteer effort and time to help a school lunch program just isn't sustainable. Although the national lunch program has the part of feeding hungry children right, it's never been well funded and has become so restricted, constricted and regulated that there's no space for healthy improvement or expansion. My conclusion is the National School Lunch Program is dead and living in the U.S.! We have the challenge and opportunity to create something new for our children. These are creative times. I am confident we will.

On the other hand, school gardens and life lab programs are growing and expanding. Funding, volunteering, and supporting educational garden programs in schools is something to get behind. Children love going to and participating in all kinds of farm and garden programs.

Sugar, fat, refined flours, HFCS, GMOs, and other unhealthy ingredients can put someone trying to live a healthy lifestyle three steps back. The refined foods practically melt in our mouths and are easy for us to eat, but very difficult for the body to digest and manage.

I continue the work of keeping that stuff to a minimum, even as I feed Savanah fruits and vegetables. Avoiding white flour, sugar and HFCS continues to be my mantra for myself, raising Savanah, and in my service with children in general. I use Stevia, honey, Agave, and fruit whenever I can get away with not using refined sugar. I try to plan and think ahead. "Savanah, you have a birthday party later today. No, you can not have sorbet at the Farmers Market." It's no fun, and sometimes painful, for me to say no.

I remember seeing a headline article on the Internet this year, which reported that refined white flour and sugar was at the top of the list for threats to kids' health. Daily I have to remind myself to do my best to keep the refined flours and sugars away. It's a huge challenge in a junk food society! All the health gurus agree that white flour and sugar wreak havoc on the body, and now we have HFCS to contend with, too.

This last Halloween I let Savanah keep ten pieces of candy and she negotiated me up to twenty pieces along with her stuffed animal toy trade for the rest of the hundred pieces of treats. I'm really uncomfortable with her eating candy, but I'm trying not to fight about it. While I worked on the computer, Savanah sat admiring the many different candy wrappers and experiencing new flavors. She bit into something, "Oh, Mom! What! This has...Just look at this!" She pushed the candy in my face so I could get a close look and asked me excitedly, "What is this, Mom?" I said, "That, Savanah, is a Snickers." I once read that Snickers was the number one best selling chocolate candy bar. And that other mom was right; Savanah did grow out of her disfavor of chocolate.

It's the middle of December and we are deep in the holiday season. Savanah has some chocolate coins. As I work on finishing this book she interrupts me, "Mom, can I eat this chocolate now?" I respond matter of fact, "Eating chocolate is a bad way to start the day. I can make you some breakfast, but if you want to eat it, go ahead." She smiled and skipped off. I feel uncomfortable watching her eat candy. At the same time, I don't want to find her hiding in the closet with any candy she is able to procure.

Not long ago I went to my family doctor for a check up and as he asked how I was doing. I offered up some complaint and then said, "But I'm not sure how serious to take me because I've read a hundred health books, and now I'm suffering from health anxiety." My doctor responded immediately, "The whole country is suffering from health anxiety." I smiled and thought how right he is.

We have a million health and cook books out now, and health topics are ubiquitous in news headlines, on the Internet and parent online groups. I also mentioned to the doctor that I was finishing up a book about feeding children. I briefly gave him a run down on the subjects n the book, and then he readily gave me his professional thoughts on what needs to be done to help our children. He said adamantly, "Put tax on fat."

The good doctor also related a story about visiting one of his relatives who was raising a small child and said he noticed bottles of empty apple juice jugs. I nodded and said, "Yes, ruins the teeth." He responded, "More than that, the child's behavior. I sat down and had a long talk with the parents and since they've cut out all that juice, the child has calmed down and is able to focus better."

As I left the doctor's office I felt more comfortable about having imposed and asking my daughter's teacher to control the sweets in her class. One of the doctor's solemn statements rang in my ears: "Save your kids now and save them from a life of sickness." As a family doctor, he understands intimately the very serious trouble our children are in today.

After the first week of the school year, I emailed Savanah's teacher about my efforts to avoid sweets whenever possible with Savanah and, to get her to take me more seriously, I mentioned Savanah's dental work. (I regularly notice the common place of silver crowns amongst her fellow school mates.) I wrote: "Do you have a general policy about sweets in the classroom? Do you limit treats to holidays? I'm concerned about a lot of birthdays on top of all the holidays."

She emailed me back. "I will bring up the topic at Back to School night. We have had one birthday so far and the crown, song, and attention was enough. We didn't have treats and nobody missed them. If treats do come, I will be sure to remind Savanah of your wishes."

With a heavy a sigh, I responded, "Just to clarify, I don't want differential treatment for Savanah. She can have whatever all the other kids are having. I guess I wrote asking for your influence over the 10% of parents who would happily not bring treats if they understood others would really appreciate it if they didn't."

All the parents gathered in the classroom for Back to School night and the teacher had their complete attention. She talked about reading, homework, and volunteers. She continued: "For birthdays, the child gets to put on the birthday crown and we sing happy birthday to them and that works just great. If you want to bring in a treat, please bring healthy birthday treats. We want the kids to stay healthy."

My jaw dropped. I was so pleased. It's her class. She makes the rules, and she just set the tone for the whole school year. Yeah! I like this word, "encouragement." It may not sound like much but it took courage for me to encourage the teacher to avoid the sweets in her classroom, and I felt so glad I did say something.

Michael brought Savanah home from a dentist appointment check up and cleaning. He got a pen flashlight and had her open her mouth for me. There, quietly hiding and growing in the back of her mouth, were the tops of her permanent molars beginning their climb. Upon seeing them I felt both a sense of the miraculous and dread. Michael said, "These next six months are critical. We need to keep these teeth clean so that we can get some sealants on top of them after they're fully in.

The dentist said to spend a minute gently cleaning, on each side." I thought how two minutes of brushing is a long time. I make a sign for myself and put it on the refrigerator: "Keep Savanah's teeth clean one day at a time." Savanah still gets giddy and twisty when it's time to brush her teeth but she cooperates. She's old enough to get it and understands. Throughout the day, when I say, "Let's brush your teeth," she acquiesces willingly.

The woman who cuts my hair is a jet set, big city bound hairdresser who is really into food, different cuisines, chefs, and cooking shows. I commented that I'm trying to figure out what to do for Thanksgiving other than turkey. She quickly countered, "It's so easy now. You can go on the Internet and find all kinds of recipes." Stunned, I quietly said, "Yeah." In my mind I thought, *It is anything but easy.* Doing the whole less meat thing, considering what constitutes proteins and a good variety of them as well as how much to make and what Savanah will eat—it's crazy hard. Feeding kids is difficult. As challenging as it is, as a global community we are making progress. We are and we have been in a food revolution. Awareness about the growing and production of food as well as the need for stronger school lunches continues to gain greater momentum.

Apart from some difficulty with her teeth, Savanah has all of them. Savanah has enjoyed good health. She is neither overweight nor underweight, has no digestive issues or allergies. She thrives well on a plant-based diet, which isn't possible for every child. I am always grateful for this. Many parents are struggling to deal with their children's food sensitivities, allergies, obesity, diabetes, asthma, things much worse than asthma such as cancer, behavioral issues, emotional and psychological issues. Many also can't get their kids to eat much in the way of whole foods. Some parents do not even have the means to give their children everything they need to thrive in perfect accordance with a healthy lifestyle—some parents do not have the time even when they try and try to make time.

I reach out to you with my heart-felt experience as one mother on a journey with her daughter through a junk food society. I wish on a star that more children can grow in their own gardens and know the deliciousness of fresh fruits and vegetables, feel their bodies grow stronger, and cultivate good habits in their children. I want people everywhere struggling to feed their children, regardless of their various schedules, anxieties, and roadblocks, to say to themselves at the end of the day, with confidence and relief, *I've done it today. I've fed my children well.*

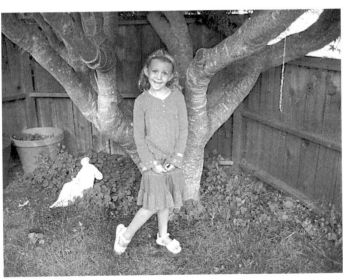

A picture of Savanah at 6-years-old under her beloved Maple tree in her garden.

Has this book been helpful?

Has this book been helpful to you and your family? If so, please consider leaving a positive review on Amazon so other parents or caregivers may be helped as well. If on the other hand, you feel there is something inside this book needs to be changed or added to in some way please send an email so those changes can be made: Sue@healhtykidshealthydiet.com

About the Author

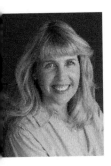

Sue Kuivanen is a credentialed secondary English teacher, who has taught children and adults of all ages. Currently she is owner of Joy and Happiness Events, an event planning company that specializes in creating and promoting health and wellness expos.

Her strong interest in the needs of children and the environment took root during her grammar school years, and she began her teaching work with Special Olympic kids throughout her high school years. College life also opened her to what were then more alternative lifestyles like yoga, vegetarianism, and various healing arts. While in college, she developed a strong desire to write a book but could never think of a compelling enough topic to undertake the commitment. After becoming a mother, Sue received the inspiration she needed to write about subjects that had been playing a predominant role in her life: health, children and the planet.

During the young years of the Internet, Sue began working as a business and IT consultant, which involved numerous gap analysis projects. More out of habit than planning, Sue approached the issue of feeding kids well by looking at the gap of what the many experts were expounding and the vastly different reality of what feeding children looks like today. Through storytelling, extensive research and field work, she provides a source of wisdom for guardians of children who would like to make conscious decisions to create happy and healthy lifestyles for their families and communities.

Sue currently lives in the Santa Cruz Mountains of California with her husband, Michael, daughter Savanah, and Australian Labradoodle, Tulip.

Her website is: www.HealthyKidsHealthyDiet.com
Email: Sue@healthykidshealhydiet.com

Get Susan's FREE report:

How to stop fighting about food with your kids.

Visit www.HealthyKidsHealthyDiet.com/freereport

BIBLIOGRAPHY

Arlin, Stephen, et al. Nature's First Law: The Raw-Food Diet. Maul Brothers Publishing, 2003.

Batmanghelidj, Fereydoon. Your Body's Many Cries for Water. 2nd ed. Detroit, MI: Global Health Solutions, 2003.

Boutenko, Victoria. 12 Steps to RAW FOODS. 1st ed. Berkeley, California: North Atlantic Books, 2007.

Cline, Foster, Jim Fay, and M. D. Parenting teens with love & logic: preparing adolescents for responsible adulthood. Colorado Springs, Colo. Pinon Press, 1992.

Campbell, Colin T., ed. The China Study. Benbella Books, 2005.

Cousens, Gabriel. Conscious Eating. 2nd ed. Berkeley, Calif. North Atantic Books, 2000.

Cousens, Gabriel. Spiritual Nutrition: Six Foundations for Spiritual Life and the Awakening of Kundalini. Berkeley, Calif. North Atlantic Books, 2005.

Enig, Mary, Dr, and Sally Fallon. Eat Fat Lose Fat. Hudson Street Press, 2005.

Esser, William L., and Ronald W. Horton. Dictionary of natural foods. Bridgeport, CT: Natural Hygiene Press, 1983.

Fallon, Sally, and Enig G. Mary. Nourishing Traditions. 2nd ed. Washington DC 20007: NewTrends Publishing, inc., 2001.

Fay, Jim. Love and logic magic for early childhood: practical parenting from birth to six years. 1st ed. Golden, Colo. Love and Logic Press, 2000.

Fay, Jim. Taking the stress out of raising great kids: journal collection years 1995 to 2000. Golden: Love and Logic Institute, 2005.

Gittleman, Ann Louise. Get the Salt Out. New York, NY: Three Rivers Press, 1996.

Gittleman, Ann Louise. Get the Sugar Out. 2nd ed. Random House, Inc, 2008.

Gittleman, Ann Louise. The Fast Track One-Day Detox Diet. Morgan Road Books, 2005.

Goodall, Jane. Harvest for Hope: A Guide to Mindful Eating. Eds. Gary McAvoy and Gail Hudson. New York: Warner Books, 2005.

Graham, Douglas. 80-10-10 Diet, The: Balancing Your Health, Your Weight, and Your Life One Luscious Bite At A Time. FoodnSport Press, 2006.

Griffith, Winter H. VITAMINS: HERBS, MINERALS, & SUPPLEMENTS. Revised. U.S.A. Fisher Books, 1998.

Huggins, Hal A. It's all in your head: the link between mercury amalgams and illness. 1st ed. Garden City Park, N.Y. Avery Pub. Group, 1993.

Kingsolver, Barbara. Animal, Vegetable, Miracle. New York, NY: HarperCollins, 2007.

Kondrot, Edward C., ed. Healing the Eye. Nutritional Research Press, 2001.

Kushi, Michio. The Book of Macrobiotics: The Universal Way of Health, Happiness, and Peace. Japan Publications, Inc., 1986.

Lair, Cynthia. Feeding the Whole Family. Revised. Moon Smile Press, 1997.

Lambert, Daphne, and Tanyia Maxted-Frost. The Organic Baby & Toddler Cokbook. Green Books Ltd, 2000.

Lapine, Missy Chase. The Sneaky Chef. Philadelphia - London: Running Press, 2007.

Levine, Susan. School Lunch Politics: The Surprising History of America's Favorite Welfare Program. Princeton, New Jersey: Princeton University Press, 2008.

Lillard, Paula Polk, and Lynn Lillard Jessen. Montessori from the start: the child at home from birth to age three. 1st ed. New York: Schocken Books, 2003.

Lillard, Paula Polk. Montessori, a modern approach. New York: Schocken Books, 1972.

Lisle, Douglas J., and Alan Goldhamer. The pleasure trap: mastering the hidden force that undermines health & happiness. Summertown, Tenn. Healthy Living Publications, 2003.

Loux, Renee. Living Cuisine. New York, NY: Avery, 2003.

McCarthy, Jenny. Louder Than Words. Penguin Group Inc., 2007.

Megre, Vladimir. Anastasia. Ed. Leonid Sharashkin. Hawaii: Ringing Cedars Press, 1996.

Nison, Paul. Raw Knowledge II: Interviews with Health Achievers. Brooklyn, New York: 343 Publishing Company, 2003.

"Nutrition, Physical Exercise, and Obesity: What's Happening in Your School? 2005/2006 Survey Results." The Center for Health and Healthcare in Schools. 28 Feb. 2008. <http://www.healthinschools.org/Publications-and-Resources/Polls-and-Surveys/Web-Based-Surveys/Nutrition-Physical-Exercise-and-Obesity-2005-2006-Survey-Results.aspx>.

Olive, Diane. Think Before You Eat: Avoid Dis-ease by Creating Better Balance and Greater Health. Glendale, California: Griffin Publishing, 1994.

Price, Weston A. Nutrition and Physical Degeneration. 6th ed. Los Angeles: Keats Publishing, 1998.

Rockwell, Sally. Coping with Candida Cookbook.0-916575-00-4. Seattle, Washington: 17th Wonderful Printing, 1996.

Rosemond, John K. The new six-point plan for raising happy, healthy children. Kansas City, Mo. Andrews McMeel Pub., 2006.

Saunders, Jeraldine, and DrHarvey Ross. Hypoglycemia The Classic Healthcare Handbook. 2nd ed. New York, NY: Kensington Publishing Corp, 2002.

Sears, William. The attachment parenting book: a commonsense guide to understanding and nurturing your baby. 1st ed. Boston: Little, Brown, 2001.

Sears, William and Martha. The Family Nutrition Book. Little, Brown & Company, 1999.

Semon, Bruce, Lori Kornblum, and Bernard Rimland. Feast without yeast: 4 stages to better health. Milwaukee, Wis. Wisconsin Institute of Nutrition, 1999.

Shelton, Herbert M., Jo Willard, and Jean A. Oswald. The Original Natural Hygiene Weight Loss Diet Book. New Canaan, Conn. Keats Publishing, 1986. 06 December 2006.

Shelton, Herbert. Fasting Can Save Your Life. Natural Hygiene Press, 1964.

Shelton, Herbert. The Science and Fine Art of Fasting. American Natural Hygiene Society, 1978.

Stoycoff, Cheryl. RAW KIDS: Transitioning Children to a Raw Diet. 2nd ed. Claremore, OK: Living Spirit Press, 2006.

Sweet, Win and Bill. Living joyfully with children. Lakewood, CO: Acropolis Books, 1997.

Ward, Janie Victoria. The Skin We're in: Teaching Our Children to Be Emotionally Strong, Socially Smart, Spiritually Connected. New York: Free Press, 2000.

Wood, Rebecca. The New Whole foods Encyclopedia. New York, NY: Penguin Compass, 1999.

Made in the USA
San Bernardino, CA
29 June 2018